Fundamental Aspects of Caring for the Person with Dementia

PS1

2

J

1 7

Other titles in the Fundamental Aspects of Nursing series include:
Adult Nursing Procedures edited by Penny Tremayne and Sam Parboteeah
Caring for the Acutely Ill Adult edited by Pauline Pratt
Community Nursing edited by John Fowler
Complementary Therapies for Health Care Professionals by Nicky Genders
Gynaecology Nursing by Sandra Johnson
Legal, Ethical and Professional Issues in Nursing by Maggie Reeves and Jacquie
    Orford
Men's Health by Morag Gray
Tissue Viability Nursing by Cheryl Dunford and Bridgit Günnewicht
Palliative Care Nursing by Robert Becker and Richard Gamlin
Women's Heath by Morag Gray

Series Editor: John Fowler

Other titles of interest:
New Ways of Working in Mental Health edited by James Dooher
Forensic Mental Health Nursing: Interventions with people with 'personality disorder'
    edited by the National Forensic Nurses' Research and Development Group
Palliative Care in Severe Dementia edited by Julian Hughes
Legal Aspects of Consent by Bridgit Dimond
Legal Aspects of Patient Confidentiality by Bridgit Dimond
Legal Aspects of Medicines by Bridgit Dimond

Note

Health care practice and knowledge are constantly changing and developing as new re-search and treatments, changes in procedures, drugs and equipment become available.

The author and publishers have, as far as is possible, taken care to confirm that the infor-mation complies with the latest standards of practice and legislation.

Fundamental Aspects of Caring for the Person with Dementia

Kirsty Beart

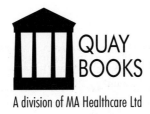

QUAY
BOOKS

A division of MA Healthcare Ltd

Quay Books Division, MA Healthcare Ltd, St Jude's Church, Dulwich Road, London SE24 0PB

British Library Cataloguing-in-Publication Data
A catalogue record is available for this book

© MA Healthcare Limited 2006

ISBN-13: 978 1 85642 303 8
ISBN-10: 1 85642 303 4

Printed by Gutenberg Press Ltd, Gudja Road, Tarxien, Malta

Contents

PART I

Theoretical information and debates, explanation, and policies of care

CHAPTER I

Imagine...

If you can, try to imagine the life you have now changing beyond all recognition. One day you wake up and don't know where you are. You ask someone near you where you are but they seem unable to understand your question. Why do they not understand – what is wrong with them? It is hard to contemplate this and fully comprehend the emotional turmoil caused by the symptoms of a dementia-type illness.

It is important to use this book as a resource for helping individuals live with dementia. This approach is in contrast to the traditional view that the devastation of this disease is all that is left of us, or the people we care for and love. It is assumed that when a person is diagnosed with dementia that their life is just one long problem and that their personality, intellect and relationship involvement will diminish unrecognisably and that we lose the ability to learn. This idea of ageing is a negative one and does little to help us live with dementia, never mind die with it! Many authors and theorists have continued to consider old age as a time in our lives when it is normal to become incapacitated. Dementia and old age have become synonymous and are inextricably linked within our modern culture. Despite this, depression is a mental illness which is much more common (Pilgrim and Rogers, 1999). Only around 2–5% of the population aged over 65 develop a dementia-type illness. Perhaps the statistics we need to look at are the links between dementia and depression. Within this group of 2–5%, there is a large increase in the numbers of people suffering from depression and anxiety. We have to ask why this might be and if there are possible triggers:

- Could be already depressed due to isolation, which is a common phenomenon for older people
- Under-stimulation, for different reasons, can induce apathy
- Feelings of a loss of control or personal autonomy can be common and linked with elder suicide
- Increased vulnerability due to physical illness and consequent depression
- Inevitable loss of spouse, roles etc.
- Ability to maintain successful relationships when younger seems to indicate less risk of becoming depressed in old age
- Effect of abuse in old age

If we accept that all these real-life issues exist for older people then we have to realise the need to try to assist them in dealing with them. This is, however, only part of the picture. The problem with dementia is that it does not only affect the old. Young people also can develop different types of dementia, including more specific ones such as Creutzfeldt–Jakob Disease, AIDS-related, Down's syndrome-related, pathology or tumours. The needs of younger people with these problems are different in many ways, but in the attitude we take to their prognosis we should consider similarities. The problem comes not just from ageist attitudes, but also from the disease approach discussed next. The need to see these people as being in need of support to cope, rather than requiring full nursing care to die, is of paramount importance in influencing how we deal with them.

Dementia is seen by society as an illness which requires medical care and support, and naturally the emphasis of care is expected to, and usually does, come from the NHS and social services. Despite this, many people still struggle with the problems on their own because of a lack of appropriate services, little awareness of support, and/or an unskilled workforce providing it. The brain disease model of the 1990s (Sayce, 2000) argues that mental illness should be seen as an illness and not as a consequence of poor morals, as it has been in the past. Despite the best intentions of this perspective to allow people with mental health problems social freedom, the down side is that the expectation associated with treatments and cures has been added on to mental illness. If a person is suffering from an illness we expect them to be at least treated, if not cured. When this idea is used with dementia the picture becomes very bleak, and the fact that there is no cure ensures an attitude of acceptance and pity. To consider the person as having gone, or being one of the 'living dead', means the loss of them as a person. However, those who are living with dementia are actually still here and able to communicate with the rest of us in some way, even if it is through smiling, crying, repeating words or pacing up and down the living room.

The social disability model argues that people with some kind of disability are not disabled by the impairment, but by the society within which they try to function. Seeing illness such as dementia as a disability within this framework can allow us to consider the plight in a different way. The person with dementia can be seen as a person and not as a disease without any hope of cure. The person's individuality can be maintained by accepting that everyone needs emotional attachment, even those who cannot clearly communicate that need. Naomi Feil (1993) introduced validation therapy, which led us into a pattern of thinking about the individual's thoughts and feelings as relevant in any situation. The carer has to learn how to interpret what the seemingly unrecognisable comments or behaviours actually mean. Kitwood (1997) discussed dementia as much more than just a medical disease. He believed that although there is a disease element to dementia it is not the only aspect, and it should never be considered in isolation. To do this would mean the loss of the ability to recognise anything other than disease, despair and loss. Kitwood argued that the ability to look at the behaviours of the individual as meaningful and to consider the effect that we, as carers, have on that behaviour allows us to communicate more effectively on the level which is needed to provide feelings of security and comfort to those we look after.

Despite this very positive slant on dementia we are still faced with the devastation that it leaves in its wake: the loss of the individual's known personality and the unpredictable nature of a new one; the feelings of frustration at not being able to remember; the feelings of fear and anxiety at the prospect of being unable to function independently; the feelings of apprehension and inadequacy as a carer in being able to cope; the frustration of being unable to provide the appropriate resource as a professional; and the inevitable anger, terror and sheer disappointment in your life's path! All of these experiences and feelings are the effects of dementia and are the reason we are here.

So, read this book with the aim of seeing the perspective of the person who has been labelled as suffering with dementia, and of the carers and professionals. Try to 'imagine' how it feels to be the other party (or indeed any of them) and then reconsider your contribution to the problems that you or they are faced with.

The book is split into two parts to help you identify the parts you need to read at different times or for varying purposes. Part 1 offers information and debate about the theoretical issues and explanations of dementia and memory loss.

Themes throughout the book include explanations of what dementia actually is and where it comes from in the first place. There are differing theories on this, and Chapter 2 establishes a basic explanation of the generally accepted definitions of dementia and its source. Learning about this helps us to understand a background to a very confusing and emotionally traumatic experience. This capacity to comprehend a little of what is going on for the person with dementia (sufferer) and the carer (professional and non-professional) can assist with developing an ability to adapt and cope with its effects, as well as influencing our reactions to the problems encountered.

Chapter 3 takes the reader into the area of finding out what people with dementia and memory problems need and want. It also considers the carer's perspective and the use of a holistic approach to caring. This involves the capacity to look at more than just a disease or any other single issue and consider the person and people involved in all aspects of their lives. Nurses, doctors, social workers, home support workers, voluntary organisation support workers, occupational therapists, physiotherapists and many more professionals are involved in caring for people with these problems, and the approaches that are discussed here in terms of assessment can be utilised by any of them with appropriate training and experience.

Establishing what the sufferer and carer need is most effective when led by an assessment strategy. This approach, however, will often be socially defined and based in cultural belief. Whilst this is not necessarily a bad thing, it does restrict people and the choices they are able to make about their own destiny.

A move towards more collaborative care approaches has meant that there has been a development in this area: helping people to live with dementia and memory problems as defined by them, rather than by the professional body and society controlling the person and their care, is the new culture in care and support.

Chapter 4 explains why this book was written in the way it was. The professional, political and ethical perspectives of care are discussed and given a background in an effort to explain the motivation of services and their ultimate goals. The interview transcripts are produced as a result of the vital collation of insight from carers and sufferers already living with dementia. This approach was taken to offer the reader insightful, understandable and practical guidance from reality to balance the professional research-based evidence of care.

Part 2 moves on to the more practical side of things. Many areas of concern for carers and professionals alike are similar. However, the experience of the problems will vary as each is influenced by the individual perspective. The reaction to problems or to living with dementia depends on this belief system. So the person with dementia or memory problems and the professional or non-professional carer can only bring their ideas and perspectives together to be able to benefit from each other.

The chapters in Part 2 consider the impact of the issues identified through the interviews as the most prominent areas. The carer's perspective is considered in conjunction with the sufferer's and a perspective on coping skills is offered. This expert teaching by those living with these problems is enhanced by evidence and research intermittently, but essentially is aimed at a combined approach of non-professional and professional carers using their own expertise to create quality care. All the text following is based on the assumption that this is a useful collaboration and that the learning points – 'How can we help ourselves and each other?' – are meant for professionals and non-professionals alike. All of the quoted text comes from the comments made by the respondents in Chapter 4. In this part they are broken down into themes and considered in more depth.

Chapter 5 begins with the psychological and emotional issues associated with dementia and memory loss. Identified areas of concern focus on the fear of dementia, personality changes, change in relationships, carer stress, and safety or rational risk.

Chapter 6 considers the support needed by carers and the support which can be offered by professionals. It introduces some legal concepts and issues, which services are generally available and the use of a collaborative approach to areas such as younger people with these problems. The use of medication and technology is also addressed as a support strategy and ends with a list of agencies actively engaged in supporting people with memory problems and dementia and their carers.

Chapter 7 begins to consider the day-to-day problems of life with dementia and memory loss. The loss of the ability to communicate and function in activities which were once commonplace can be very distressing and difficult to accommodate. The chapter looks at household tasks and how to deal with loss of skill whilst balancing the need to maintain ability and dignity with safety. The personal care abilities of an individual are very seriously affected by memory loss and are included here to demonstrate this as well as to show the ways in which self-care skills – hygiene, sleep, using the toilet, eating and drinking, preventing skin damage and monitoring pain – can be part of the daily routine. Social lives often fall victim to the disturbing affects of dementia and people find it very awkward to maintain a social life at all. The general principles demonstrated in this chapter can help to ensure that people with dementia and carers are aware that this option is not automatically closed down.

The final chapter discusses thinking and the effect that disturbances like memory loss and dementia can have on a person's ability to continue with their normal intellectual processes in daily life. Communication is affected and the chapter offers some insight into understanding what this means for the individual. Examples of the use of therapeutic approaches indicate how to cope with these problems and include descriptions of the use of approaches such as validation therapy, resolution therapy, positive person work and psychosocial interventions, as well as other well-known interventions used by professionals. The context of the writing is not to teach the person to be a therapist, but simply to identify and explore the potential use of these and their underlying philosophies of care in the approach offered by the carer.

References

Feil, N. (1993) *The Validation Breakthrough: Simple Techniques for Communicating with People with Dementia*. Health Professions Press, London.

Kitwood, T. (1997) *Dementia Reconsidered: The Person Comes First*. Open University Press, Buckingham.

Pilgrim, D. and Rogers, A. (1999) *A Sociology of Mental Health and Illness*, 2nd edn. Open University Press, Buckingham.

Sayce, L. (2000) *From Psychiatric Patient to Citizen – Overcoming Discrimination and Social Exclusion*. Macmillan Press, London.

CHAPTER 2

What it means to have symptoms of dementia and memory loss

Learning points on dominant explanations of dementia:

- Understanding the relevance of theoretical definitions and the ways in which they affect a person living with dementia
- Social definitions and their implications
- Medical explanations and the evidence for disease models with a chemical/ biological basis
- Alternative theories of dementia, including social and learned behaviour debates

The standard descriptions available of what dementia actually is usually focus on its medical diagnosis and treatment. These may include definitions such as a 'syndrome characterised by loss of intellectual capacity in multiple domains' (Henderson, 1994). Despite this there is often a difference in how people with dementia, their carers and professionals identify, label and prioritise the symptoms (Garland and Hall, 2000). Many professionals will define the illness by the deterioration of cognitive abilities (brain function), whilst sufferers and carers will refer to behavioural problems. It is important to understand the need to classify an illness so that appropriate research can take place in an effort to develop treatment and care strategies. Much research is being undertaken into the causes and treatment of different types of dementia, and some progress has been made with the introduction of medications called 'acetylcholinesterase inhibitors', like Aricept and Exelon. These drugs have shown some benefit in slowing down the process in clinical trials, but overall they have a limited benefit and are not a cure.

Social definitions

Despite the need for classification and labelling, these can in themselves be quite limiting and even potentially dangerous to the individuals involved. This sounds very dramatic, but the issues around disease and labelling are very important to the way we view and attend to certain problems like dementia. For example, as a society we very much link dementia with old age, despite depression being the most common illness in the older population, whilst dementia occurs in only 5–6% of the total population over 65 years old (Pilgrim and Rogers, 1999). This particular labelling of older people and people with dementia can influence how we value the part these groups of people play in society, and consequently how much they are allowed to make their own decisions.

During the 1990s there was a common theme in health care which viewed mental illness as a disease of the brain which is no different from disease in any organ of the body (Sayce, 2000). This idea seems very appealing, as it offers us a means of trying to fix the problem, and indeed that is what it did for dementia. The growth of research into dementia has continued and escalated. The idea that mental illness is neither a moral weakness, nor the fault of parents or environment, also removes the element of blame, which can often mean feelings of guilt compounding the problem for those concerned. The problem is that this means that responsibility for the person's own destiny is defined by others. People with dementia and their carers' views can easily be ignored, as they are not expert clinicians. The lack of definition by the medical model of dementia is obvious when we remind ourselves that a clear pathological diagnosis is not actually clear at all. Most of the diagnosis depends on inappropriate behaviours which lead to a disease diagnosis; the link between the two is vague and unconvincing. The contradiction lies in the fact that the medical model defines it as an organic illness, and yet the evidence of the link between organic damage and the associated symptoms is unreliable. Many people have organic damage and no dementia. An example of this concern lies in the research that has considered language ability to be an area of decline associated with age; however, it remains a diagnostic tool for identifying and measuring dementia (Harding and Palfrey, 1997). If older people already have a natural change or decline in this area, then the question should be why is this not seen as normal ageing?

The debate about how to define mental illness has gone on for many years, and dementia is included within it. This means that when people have dementia they depend on the help of people who may have different views. Some authors, like Szasz (1987; cited in Bowers, 1998), have claimed that mental illness is a metaphysical phase and that all illnesses are physiological malfunctions or not illnesses at all, while Sedgwick (1982; cited in Bowers, 1998) said that all illnesses are socially defined, suggesting that there are no illnesses or disease in society. The person usually accesses medical treatment, as dementia is seen as a disease, looking for help with expectations of cure and treatment. The reality is that we do not have a cure for this illness and most support offered is focused on helping people to live with the problems they are faced with.

Still there is no agreed definition of how to define mental illness and the particular disorders which come under its umbrella, such as dementia. The use of diagnoses and characteristics does offer us a means of identifying certain patterns and helping each other to cope. It is possible to come together as a group of individuals trying to help in the enormously complex situation of living with dementia.

Whilst it is important to continue with this aspect of research and development, looking for treatments, cures and prevention strategies, it needs to be remembered that meanwhile there are already people in our communities, hospitals and lives living with dementia, and they need help to continue doing so.

Therefore this book will talk about the nature of understanding what it means to have dementia and how informal carers and professional carers alike can develop skills in helping people to live with dementia.

What else should we consider?

The problem with limiting a diagnosis to a loss of cognitive ability is that it misses out the other important elements of the symptoms and therefore support required. Whilst in itself using a diagnosis is not a problem, it becomes so when the carers and professionals get together to plan the future. Despite this, it is possible to gain cross-awareness through the use of carer and professional education about each other's perspective. The use of relationship-centred care (Nolan *et al.*, 2001) may well enhance this notion, as it considers the benefits of a combination approach. This method considers the need to examine the dynamic of all the people involved in the situation which arises from a person having symptoms of dementia. In the process of considering the need for greater use of combined carer/client perspectives there is also an urgent need to recognise the responsibilities of the professionals in moving forward with this theme also. There is a potential need for generic health workers with specific care skills, the involvement of families and the more effective use of available services. The current development of the Ten Essential Shared Capabilities (Hope, 2004; see box), is perhaps the beginning of instituting this idea in mental health care, and then more specifically of introducing it to the care of people with dementia.

How big is this problem for society?

Alzheimer's Disease International (2000), cited in Norman and Ryrie (2004), state that in the year 2000, 18 million people had a diagnosis of dementia. The Alzheimer's Society (2000) identify that in the UK 800,000 people are diag-

The Ten Essential Shared Capabilities for mental health practice (Hope, 2004)

Working in partnership	Developing and maintaining constructive working relationships with service users, carers, families, colleagues, lay people and wider community networks. Working positively with any tensions created by conflicts of interest or aspiration that may arise between the partners in care.
Respecting diversity	Working in partnership with service users, carers, families and colleagues to provide care and interventions that not only make a positive difference but also do so in ways that respect and value diversity, including age, race, culture, disability, gender, spirituality and sexuality.
Practising ethically	Recognising the rights and aspirations of service users and their families, acknowledging power differentials and minimising them whenever possible. Providing treatment and care that is accountable to service users and carers within the boundaries prescribed by national (professional), legal and local codes of ethical practice.
Challenging inequality	Addressing the causes and consequences of stigma, discrimination, social inequality and exclusion for service users, carers and mental health services. Creating, developing or maintaining valued social roles for people in the communities they come from.
Promoting recovery	Working in partnership to provide care and treatment that enable service users and carers to tackle mental health problems with hope and optimism and to work towards a valued lifestyle within and beyond the limits of any mental health problem.
Identifying people's needs and strengths	Working in partnership to gather information to agree health and social care needs in the context of the preferred lifestyle and aspirations of service users their families, carers and friends.
Providing service user-centred care	Negotiating achievable and meaningful goals; primarily from the perspective of service users and their families. Influencing and seeking the means to achieve these goals and clarifying the responsibilities of the people who will provide any help that is needed, including systematically evaluating outcomes and achievements.
Making a difference	Facilitating access to and delivering the best quality, evidence-based, values-based health and social care interventions to meet the needs and aspirations of service users and their families and carers.

Promoting safety and positive risk taking	Empowering the person to decide the level of risk they are prepared to take with their health and safety. This includes working with the tension between promoting safety and positive risk taking, including assessing and dealing with possible risks for service users, carers, family members and the wider public.
Personal development and learning	Keeping up-to-date with changes in practice and participating in life-long learning and personal and professional development for one's self and colleagues through supervision, appraisal and reflective practice.

nosed with the condition. As the UK has an ageing population they estimate that these numbers will rise because ageing is a key risk factor in the onset of dementia. By 2050 it is expected that 1.2 million people will have this diagnosis Department of Health (2001). The figures highlight an enormous issue for service provision. The need to plan well is paramount, especially given these projections, and the only way to even get close to the appropriate way forward is through the combined approach identified here.

There are many ways of describing how dementia affects people in their everyday lives. We are constantly hearing reference to becoming 'senile' or 'demented' in common language. The use of these terms can be misleading when we realise that *senile* simply means *old*, and dementia is a degenerative disease which is much more serious than a glib reference to memory loss. With this in mind it is important to understand that young people get dementia too, and people who have dementia may not find their diagnosis or problems very funny. This person (Alzheimer's Society, 2004a) gives a very powerful analogy of just how the disease affected her and allows us to see the anguish of the person with the problem from their perspective:

> To me, it's like knitting with a knotted ball of wool. Every now and then I come to a knot. I try to unravel it but can't, so I knit the knot in. As time goes by, there are more and more knots.

Medical explanation of dementia

Dementia is a syndrome due to disease of the brain, usually of chronic or progressive nature, in which there is a disturbance of multiple higher cortical functions. (Henderson, 1994)

The areas affected by the illness include learning and memory, language, behaviour, emotions, social interaction and abilities in day-to-day life skills.

Although there is a common umbrella term of *dementia*, there are many types which have different possible/unknown causes, symptoms and treatments/care. As a result of being able to differentiate between them, individuals can be offered much more effective support which targets the disease process that they are experiencing. Despite this diagnostic separation of types, recent research has begun to consider commonalities between some of them and their pathology in the brain. There is an assertion that a combination of Alzheimer's and vascular types are linked to each other, and that this is more common in older people's dementia (Skoog, 2004). This kind of research is based on the premise that many people who have either type of change in the brain often have the other as well. To explain: a person with vascular dementia will be seen to have damaged areas in the brain due to oxygen deprivation and those with Alzheimer's will have small protein bodies causing cell death. In the absolute diagnosis (which only occurs after death), some people have been found to have both pathologies and yet they only displayed symptoms of either vascular or Alzheimer's dementia.

Table 2.1 identifies some of the more commonly known types of dementia with a summary of key symptoms and medical interventions. This is not an exhaustive list, and many of the symptoms are similar in each. Many of the treatments are still being investigated with regard to their effectiveness for the different problems.

As Table 2.1 shows, the majority of people are diagnosed with one of the types of dementia identified. However, there are around 5% of people who develop different dementia processes (Alzheimer's Society, 2004b), and these are listed in Table 2.2.

The last category of dementia types is those that occur as a result of other problems and they are described in Table 2.3.

The diagnosis of dementia (Figure 2.1) is made as a result of medical examinations. This may include memory tests etc., but will ultimately involve a lot of physical testing to exclude any other cause of the symptoms. If nothing else is found then dementia can be considered a viable diagnosis.

Alternative views of dementia

If the humanistic perspective is to be believed then the care of people with dementia becomes much more focused on the person's identity rather than on their illness.

Table 2.1 Common types of dementia and their treatment.

Diagnosis	Common symptoms	Treatments
Mild cognitive impairment		
■ Commonly known as a transition phase between normal ageing and dementia ■ 5–15% convert to Alzheimer's Disease (AD) within 1 year (Feldman *et al.*, 2004) ■ 50% will convert to AD in 3–4 years (Hanninen *et al.*, 2004)	Memory loss is the main issue; much less decline of other brain functions (Antuono, 2004). Reduced concentration and dexterity, and consequently functioning skill Depression and anxiety are more common if the client is older (Hanninen *et al.*, 2004), and if they have poor cognitive (brain function, e.g. thinking) ability (Tschanz *et al.*, 2004; Mathuranath *et al.*, 2004).	Donepezil and certain vitamins have the potential to be used to reduce risk of progression to AD.
Alzheimer's Disease		
■ 55% of people with dementia have AD (Alzheimer's Society, 2004) ■ Severe brain cell loss linked to finding of plaques and tangles of protein in the brain ■ However, these proteins are found in people without AD (Alzheimer's Society, 2005)	Memory loss, intellectual decline, behavioural changes, functional ability loss All symptoms vary and are usually gradual Death will usually occur due to other illness, e.g. chest infections, pneumonia. The course of the AD could be as much as 15 years	Anti-cholinesterase Inhibitors (e.g. Aricept, Exelon) Memantine Some of these drugs are not available, but they and many more are being researched for their usefulness. So far evidence has suggested some benefits to carers and clients through the reduction of difficult behaviours (Winblad, 2004), but they are not a cure.
Multi-infarct/vascular type dementia		
■ 20% of people with dementia have vascular dementia (Alzheimer's Society, 2004) ■ Brain is deprived of oxygen ■ Caused by massive numbers of tiny strokes or one major stroke, or by Binswanger's Disease (severe damage to the white matter of the brain caused by hypertension – high blood pressure). Binswanger's Disease is very rare.	Similar symptoms to Alzheimer's Disease, but the onset may be more sporadic and sudden. The progression of this type tends to be in stages, as the damage occurs in stages.	Reduction of risk of vascular disease is a key area in prevention. After onset, anti-oxidant, anti-inflammatory drugs may have an impact in slowing the process down. Again, these are not cures.

Table 2.1 (continued)

Lewy body dementia		
■ 15–20% of people with dementia have Lewy body dementia (Ballard, 2004) ■ Protein deposits on nerve cells which disrupt normal brain function ■ However, the proteins are found in many people without the illness	Fluctuating cognitive ability; visual-spatial and perceptual disturbance; falls or loss of consciousness; loss of self-care skills	Anti-Parkinsonian drugs, which reduce the disturbing symptoms Anti-cholinesterase (Aricept, Exelon) drugs are being researched as to their use for this group.

Within this theoretical perspective there is a need to assume that people (Rogers, 1961):

■ Are generally OK and not bad, but may need help to recognise that fact.
■ Can discover their own meanings, but may need help doing so.
■ Know what they need, but may need help expressing it.
■ Take responsibility for themselves, but may need encouragement to do so.

If carers (professional or non-professional) can achieve this level of acceptance and release themselves from taking complete control, then the potential for developing 'personhood' (Kitwood, 1997) and learning to cope with dementia is expected to become less stressful and more supportive.

The concerns of many people may relate to the lack of awareness that most individuals with dementia have. Disorientation can lead to becoming lost; forgetting names and places can lead to frustration and becoming vulnerable; and generally a loss of control of self-care tasks can result in poor hygiene and physical health. All of these problems and many more lead us to assume that when a person has dementia they immediately lose the capacity to make decisions or look after any aspect of their day-to-day lives. Perhaps the issue here is not about overall ability but about individual progress and deterioration of skills. For example, a person in the latter stages of dementia may be unable to hold a clear conversation using the appropriate words. As a result, it is often assumed that they cannot communicate their thoughts or ideas, and may not have any in the first place. Many therapeutic approaches reject this notion and suggest that any words spoken by a person with dementia have significance: validation therapy is an example (Feil, 1993; Kitwood, 1997). Both Feil and Kitwood are significant proponents of person-centred theories and their ideas promote the notion that the carer can learn what the seemingly nonsensical conversation of the person with dementia actually means and therefore promote the ideas of the humanistic perspective. The person is trying to tell you something, but it is not easy to understand because of their speech problems. This is not the same as not knowing what they want. A person who is unable to communicate verbally that

Table 2.2 Less common dementias.

Diagnosis	Symptoms	Treatment
Human prion disease ■ Creutzfeldt–Jakob Disease (CJD): damage-causing proteins which cause brain to become soft and spongy ■ Sporadic; 85% of all cases have unknown cause ■ Iatrogenic: 10–15% of all cases. Caused by direct infection of person, e.g. by surgery ■ Familial: 10–15% of all cases have genetic links ■ Variant CJD linked to Bovine Spongiform Encephalopathy (BSE); and holds risk for young people. Numbers have varied annually due to suspected cases increasing around 1998–2003. Since and before this time definite diagnosis cases are small in number (National CJD Surveillance Unit, 2005).	Sudden onset and usually quick progression. Starts with memory lapses and mood changes. Clumsiness, feeling muddled, slurred speech and jerky movements/falling over. Final stages are usually within 6 months to 2 years and include severe disability and loss of independence.	Currently no treatment is available. Some trials are under way considering the effects of three main types of drug: quinacrine, pentosan polysulphate and flupirtine. All of these have had some success in trials with animals and even some positive effects on clinically ill patients, but none have demonstrated clear evidence of benefits yet. Potential benefits are about slowing down or halting the process of CJD in clinically diagnosed patients (National CJD Surveillance Unit, 2005)
Huntington's Disease ■ Genetic disorder which begins at around 30 –40 years old (Alzheimer's Society, 2005) ■ 50–50 chance of children taking faulty gene from parent (Huntington's Disease Association, 2005)	Reduced ability to carry out planning or to organise self and life. Loss of memory; speech and swallowing problems; lack insight; clumsiness and obsessive behaviours. However, people with this illness can often recognise people and places they know, which differs from other types (Alzheimer's Society, 2005).	No current treatment available Treat and care for symptoms

Table 2.2 (continued)

Korsakoff's Syndrome

▪ Caused by a combination of a severe lack of vitamin B1 (thiamine) due to poor diet and an excess intake of alcohol reducing ability to absorb nutrients ▪ Damage occurs after 10 years of this lifestyle in women/20 years in men (Alzheimer's Society, 2005)	Affects a large part of the brain; therefore symptoms are very generalised: poor learning ability; lack of insight; inventing responses to cover up gaps in memory (confabulation); apathy; long-term memory loss.	Not drinking alcohol and intensive vitamin B1 therapy can induce an improvement (Alzheimer's Society, 2005)

Wernicke's encephalopathy

▪ A transitional stage before Korsakoff's which can be reversed	Involuntary jerky movements; poor balance/walking; drowsiness; and confusion	Stopping drinking alcohol and intensive vitamin B1 therapy usually reverses process

Frontal-temporal lobe (Pick's disease)

▪ 5% of dementias (Alzheimer's Society, 2004) ▪ Damage affects specific part of brain which controls behaviour, language and emotion ▪ More likely in younger people (Alzheimer's Society, 2005)	Language problems: not finding right words; reduced involvement in conversation Personality and behaviour changes: lack insight, inappropriate behaviour and aggression Changes in eating habits	Anti-cholinesterase inhibitors make symptoms worse. No other treatment available. Speech therapy has some use.

they don't want the carer to feed them a particular food may be expressing this by crying, shouting or making one-word outbursts, for example. The point here is that the person needs to be understood rather than having their behaviour seen as inappropriate, aggressive or difficult.

The Rogerian principles of person-centred theories have been utilised heavily here and it is apparent in many carers' and professionals' approaches that this is indeed a more humane means of helping people who are having to deal with the impact of dementia on their lives.

Rogers (1967) claims that person-centred approaches depend on the willingness of carers to develop the necessary growth relationship with the person. This requires a strong level of confidence in the person's abilities and the ability of the carer to give up some of the control that they have over that person.

Rogers explains that behaviour is to a large extent an acting out of the way we actually feel about ourselves and the world we live in, and is often a reflec-

Table 2.3 Dementia caused by other diseases.

Original illness/problem	Dementia
Acquired Immune Deficiency Syndrome – AIDS	Caused by a direct impact of the HIV infection on the brain and by reduced immunity to other infections.
	Symptoms include jerky eye movements, mood swings and hallucinations (Alzheimer's Society, 2005).
	Due to the success of combination therapy for HIV, there could be a stopping or slowing down of this type of dementia.
Parkinson's Disease	Risk of developing dementia six times more than in general population. Higher risk within this group if Lewy body proteins are in the brain. People often experience hallucinations, loss of self-care skills and stiffness (Alzheimer's Society, 2005). Use of anti-cholinergics (Aricept, Exelon) is being researched.
	15–20% of people with Parkinson's will develop dementia (Parkinson's Disease Society, 2005).
Learning disability	People who have a learning disability are four times more likely to develop dementia than those without (Alzheimer's Society, 2005).
Down's Syndrome	People with Down's Syndrome have an even higher risk of developing dementia. Many develop the plaques and tangles of Alzheimer's but do not all develop the disease (Alzheimer's Society, 2005). 36% of 50–59 year-olds and 54.5% of 60–69 year-olds will develop dementia (Foundation for People with Learning Disabilities, 2001).
Multiple sclerosis	Sufferers can develop cognitive problems and dementia and this often affects concentration and memory. Research centres around use of anti-dementia drugs (Aricept etc.), and early diagnosis in helping people cope (Silber, 2005).
Thyroid deficiency/vitamin deficiency	Severe deprivation can result in dementia and there is commonly a slowing down and loss of interest in things (Alzheimer's Society, 2005).
Progressive supranuclear-palsy	Dementia onset includes visual problems (Alzheimer's Society, 2005)
Normal pressure hydrocephalus	Caused by head injury, meningitis and encephalitis (infection in the brain), which in turn obstruct the normal flow of the spinal fluid. The result can be dementia, and common symptoms include problems walking and incontinence (Alzheimer's Society, 2005)
Type C Niemann–Pick Disease	Occurs in children and adolescents; loss of movement and swallowing ability.
	If dementia occurs it can include reduced memory, concentration and learning (Alzheimer's Society, 2005).

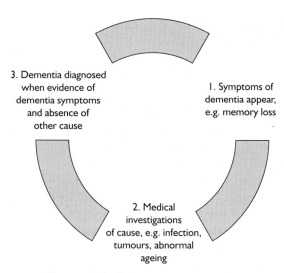

Figure 2.1 Diagnosing dementia.

tion of how we evaluate ourselves. If this is assumed to be true, then the caring person has to be able to accept that the person with dementia can be self-determining in some aspects of life, although they may need help with others.

Watkins (2001) also discusses the use of a person-centred approach in assessing people with problems. The author states:

> gathering information and understandings about a client's inner and outer worlds from their frame of reference

is beneficial to both the person with dementia and to the carer in terms of accuracy of information. Watkins claims that this approach in assessment of a person with dementia will result in enlightening both the carer and the sufferer, providing an ongoing assessment method. This will encourage a deeper understanding of a person's feelings, providing them with help to explore their own feelings, focus on strengths and not problems as usual, and explore how to cope with their life and issues more resourcefully, whilst maintaining the individual's connection between their thoughts and feelings and their actions (Watkins, 2001).

Without this approach to assessment it is almost impossible to consider an accurate assessment of people who live their lives outside of the expected British public social rules. For example, cultural differences in perspectives of life can mean that a person with dementia from a particular ethnic background may refuse personal care, as it is deemed appropriate by the professional assessor. A person of the Hindu faith may refuse personal care, as they have necessary cleansing procedures which cannot be or are not being attended to properly by a carer, etc. A person who has a non-English first language may find it very difficult to be understood, even if their speech is unaffected by the dementia. A person whose sexual orientation is not heterosexual may find that the person they have chosen to be their advocate is not recognised by the statutory rules of care in British law. All of these groups will have similar needs and wants as do those who fit our very structured and socially controlling approach to health and social care. The lack of flexibility in these issues is yet to be tackled by the services, although attempts have been made to make a person's individuality more important, and the emergence of the Mental Capacity Act 2005 promotes this and develops the concept further.

As with any theoretical ideal there are problems. The emphasis on learning to live with dementia could actually imply the lack of a need to challenge it in medical research. It must not be forgotten that medical research is making progress in identifying risk factors for developing the problem and developing medication to help ease the distress of the symptoms. Harding and Palfrey (1997) claim that the person-centred approach to dementia care is flawed, with unclear symptom patterns and ambiguity in its definition. The claim is that Kitwood in particular makes many assumptions about what is necessary for the human connection with each other and makes little attempt to justify why maintaining well-being is of benefit to anyone, never mind a person with dementia. The individual need is different in different people and to assume that all old people need the same kind of approach and respond negatively to malignant social psychology is short-sighted. The main irony lies in the rejection by Kitwood of the biomedical model because of its disease-labelling negative stereotyping and his own defining of inappropriate behaviour which needs therapising. This in itself makes the experience of dementia an illness for which people need professional care.

Another issue which is particularly prominent in a person-centred approach lies in the ability of the assessor to commit to the ideals and therefore give up some control. Carers may feel that to do so would put the person with dementia's safety or health in danger. This is a real concern and is based in the nurturing and protective aspect of the caring role.

Lastly, the person assessing may be limited in their interviewing skills or be too emotionally involved to be objective, resulting in an inappropriate approach. The problem with this is that the person being assessed may withdraw themselves emotionally and physically as they may feel threatened.

The attachment theory of Bowlby identifies a need to protect each other from danger (Tibbs, 2004), and this is an admirable and necessary aspect of care. However, it is important to remember that the individual remains here and has not become a child again or died. The personality and emotions and recognisable characteristics may have changed, but the person remains and their need for attachment remains also. The needs we all have for belonging and security and expression are essential to human existence, and people with dementia are not suddenly exempt from this need.

A last explanation of dementia lies in the social constructionist view. This is a sociological view of the world based on the assumption that the world we live in is constructed by society based on the meanings and values we place on things and events. Thus, understanding the meaning of what we do and why we do it requires us to understand how and what we created by considering what individuals' daily life activities mean. Within this tradition there is much criticism of biomedical and person-centred explanations and treatments of dementia. The social constructionist view of dementia focuses on the need of society to believe that we can find a cure for our ailments; therefore we must define all scary changes in our lives as abnormal. The need to see the development of an older person becoming old graciously is something we crave because the alternative is too horrible to consider – that it is indeed part of normal ageing to exhibit any behavioural symptoms, whether they are socially acceptable or not.

Therefore if society defines the disturbing behaviours of dementia as an illness then it is possible that there may be a cure for ageing and even death.

The theory continues that the older person has a reaction to being marginalised into a group of people who are old and therefore potentially 'demented'. The reaction could be explained in three ways as follows (Harding and Palfrey, 1997):

- The ageing brain separates itself and thus forgets how to carry out tasks.
- The rejection of the ageing body can lead to retreat from oneself, causing isolation and consequent loss of a sense of the self.
- The person exhibiting all the socially unacceptable behaviours does so because they have thrown off the shackles of social control.

Essentially, the classification of all deviant behaviour in old age as a disease called dementia is inaccurate and misleading if we consider individual meaning as significant. Harding and Palfrey (1997) adopt the ideas of Fleck's 'comparative epistemology': that there is no need for one big all-encompassing approach to dementia, but rather that there are many different types of behaviour which are socially divergent and seen in the true individual meaning of the person's context.

The concerns with this idea are that there is little attempt to understand why there are indeed patterns to behaviours exhibited by different people and that only a small number of the population actually do develop the behaviours to a severe level. Why do only some people reject the ageing body if it is part of the social construct within which we all live? Also, this view of dementia as merely a social construct implies the need to regard it as normal and therefore assume that it is not distressing. It is possibly a paradoxical effect of the theory itself that people fear the onset of old age and therefore do become very distressed by its onset and symptoms. Therefore people will crave answers, and in the Western world of developing technology it is almost an assumption that professions such as medicine will continue to look for answers and some relief.

It is perhaps true that it is a normal part of ageing to develop socially unacceptable behaviours, and it is also possibly true that there is nothing that medicine or care can do to change that. However, another condition of humankind is the need to develop itself and overcome things that it defines as distressing, and to do that with hope of our survival.

What does it all mean?

The fact is that many carers and people who have these disturbing behaviours become very distressed by its impact on their lives, and the reasons for its existence are not important to those living with it today. This is not to say that continued research for future generations into explanations should not take place, but rather that the emphasis of need is also important for those who are currently living with the issues.

The humanistic tradition has many benefits and problems when applied in the care of people with dementia. However, it does seem to offer some hope to the many people who already have these problems in their lives. The ability to see a person as an individual who needs assistance and help is often the condition needed to balance the medical intervention with maintaining the individuality and meaning of a person's life during very trying times.

References

Alzheimer's Disease International (2000) World Alzheimer's Day Bulletin. Alzheimer's Disease International, London (http://www.alzheimers.org. uk/).

Alzheimer's Society (2000) *Introduction to Dementia*. Alzheimers Society, London.

Alzheimer's Society (2004a) *What dementia feels like*. http://www.alzheimers.org.uk/Real_lives/People_with_dementia/What_dementia_feels_like/index.htm

Alzheimer's Society (2004b) *Facts about Dementia*. http://www.alzheimers.org.uk/facts-about-dementia.

Alzheimer's Society (2004c) *Real Lives.* http://www.alzheimers.org/real-lives/people-with-dementia/index.htm.

Antuono, P., Jones, J., Shi-Jiang, L., Franszak, M. and Hammeke, T. (2004) Neuropsychological measures to distinguish mild cognitive impairment from normal aging. *Neurobiology of Aging,* **25**(Supp 2), 22.

Ballard, C. (2004) Dementia with Lewy bodies: update definition and clinical studies. *Neurobiology of Aging,* **25**(Supp 2), 50–1.

Bowers, L. (1998) *The Social Nature of Mental Illness.* Routledge, London.

Caputo, M., Sebastini, V., Monastero, R., Mariani, E., Senin, U. and Mecocci, P. (2004) Behavioural and psychological symptoms in dementia: a population based study. *Neurobiology of Aging,* **25**(Supp 2), 99.

Department of Health (2001) *National Service Frameworks for Mental Health: Modern Standards and Service Models.* HMSO, London.

Feldman, H., Schelte, P., Scarpini, E., Mancioni, L. and Lane, R. (2004) Operational criteria for confirmation of clinical diagnosis of Alzheimer's disease in patients with mild cognitive impairment. *Neurobiology of Aging,* **25**(Supp 2), 472.

Feil, N. (1993) *The Validation Breakthrough: Simple Techniques for Communicating with People with Dementia.* Health Professions Press, London.

Foundation for People with Learning Disabilities (2001) *Down's Syndrome and Dementia: Briefing for Commissioners.* http://www.learningdisabilities.org.uk/page.cfm.

Garland, L. and Hall, G. R. (2000) The biological basis of behavioural symptoms in dementia. *Issues in Mental Health Nursing,* **21**, 91–107.

Hanninen, T., Hallikainen, M., Vanhanen, M. and Soininen, H. (2004) Prevalence of mild cognitive impairment: a population based study in elderly subjects. Conference poster presentation, *9th International Conference on Alzheimer's Disease and Related Disorders,* Philadelphia.

Harding, N. and Palfrey, C. (1997) *The Social Construction of Dementia: Confused Professionals.* Jessica Kingsley, London.

Henderson, A. S. (1994) *Dementia: Epidemiology of Mental Disorders.* World Health Organization, Geneva.

Hope, R. (2004) *The Ten Essential Shared Capabilities.* HMSO, London.

Huntington's Disease Association (2005) *What is Huntington's Disease?* http://www.hda.org.uk/.

Jee, M. and Reason, L. (2000) *Who Cares? Information and Support for the Carers of People with Dementia.* HMSO, London.

Kitwood, T. (1997) *Dementia Reconsidered: the Person Comes First.* Open University Press, Buckingham.

Mathuranath, P. S., Suresh Kumar, M., Mathew, R., George, A. and Cherian, J. P. (2004) Role of subjective memory complaints in defining mild cognitive impairment. *Neurobiology of Aging*, **25**(Supp 2), 74.

National Creutzfeldt–Jakob Disease Surveillance Unit (2005) http://www.cjd.ed.ac.uk/.

Nolan, M., Keady, J. and Aveyard, B. (2001) Relationship-centred care is the next logical step. *British Journal of Nursing*, **10**(12), 757.

Norman, I. and Ryrie, I. (2004) *The Art and Science of Mental Health Nursing: a Textbook of Principles and Practice*. Open University Press, New York.

Parkinson's Disease Society (2005) *Dementia and Parkinson's*. Information Sheet FS58. http://www.parkinsons.org.uk/shared_asp_files/uploadedfiles/%7BA4B3BFD5-7E51-44C5-AA8B-9D129AD2B0CA%7D_dementia5803_04.pdf

Peterson, R., Grundman, M., Thomas, R. and Thal, L. (2004) Donepezil and vitamin E as treatments for mild cognitive impairment. *Neurobiology of Aging*, **25**(Supp 2), 20.

Pilgrim, D. and Rogers, A. (1999) *A Sociology of Mental Health and Illness*, 2nd edn. Open University Press, Buckingham.

Sayce, L. (2000) *From Psychiatric Patient to Citizen – Overcoming Discrimination and Social Exclusion*. Macmillan Press, London.

Silber, E. (2005) *What can medical science offer me now? Cognition*. Multiple Sclerosis Society, London. http://www.mssociety.org.uk/search_clicks.rm?id=64&destinationtype=2&instanceid=292105.

Skoog, I. (2004) Vascular dementia: risk factors and pathophysiology. *Neurobiology of Aging*, **25**(Supp 2), 50.

Tibbs, M. A. (2004) *Social Work and Dementia: Good Practice and Care Management*. Jessica Kingsley, London.

Tschanz, J., Klein, E., Treiber, K., Corcoran, C., Norton, M., Toone, L., Welsh-Bohmer, K., Steinberg, M., Munger, R., Pieper, C., Breitner, J., Zandi, P. and Lyketsos, C. (2004) Neurospychiatric symptoms in mild cognitive impairment and dementia: prevalence and relationship to cognition and functional impairment. *Neurobiology of Aging*, **25**(Supp 2), 314.

Watkins, P. (2001) *Mental Health Nursing: the Art of Compassionate Care*. Butterworth-Heineman, Oxford.

Winblad, B. (2004) Treatments for severe Alzheimer's Disease. *Neurobiology of Aging*, **25**(Supp 2), 92.

CHAPTER 3

How we know what the person with dementia wants or needs

Learning points on how we know what a person needs:

▪ Use of assessment methods and their issues
▪ Influence of social views on the care provided
▪ Professional policy and guidelines impact on assessment
▪ Strategies for a person-centred approach
▪ Strategies for non-professional carers to offer person-centred care

The standard means of finding out if someone has dementia is through assessment. This process is influenced by professional training and social perspectives of how to care for someone in a safe and ethical way.

One of the hardest things for any carer, professional or sufferer to do is to identify the things that are needed or wanted in this ever-changing situation.

The person with dementia may have many problems, and often these are not identified even when using professional measurement scales like the Mini Mental State (Folstein et al., 1975), Neuropsychiatric Inventory (Cummings *et al.*, 1994), the Cognitive Profile (Bolland *et al.*, 1996), the Modified Mini-Cog (Borson *et al.*, 2000), CAMDEX-R (Roth *et al.*, 1998). All of these tests allow professionals to measure the functioning of a person's cognitive and functional ability, thus offering them a basis upon which to intervene.

For example, the use of the Mini Mental State is a standard measure within memory clinics used by assessors to monitor a person's progress through the problems. With this signposting it is easier for professionals to target key areas of need and then assist the sufferer and carer to access appropriate services. The use of medications like Aricept or Exelon is also prescribed based on this assessment of the severity of the illness.

The use of these tools has a place in the diagnosis and monitoring of the severity of symptoms. However, it only seems to cover essential need and illness perspectives.

There are indeed other issues which in some situations could be considered even more important. The issues of social awareness and activity are vital to the person being able to continue with social contact of any kind. This can be seen as integral to their interactions in therapeutic as well as social situations. Also, the person's psychological or mood state is important in determining the impact that this will have on functioning and the potential onset of depression: 10–15% of people over 65 suffer from depression (Department of Health, 2001). For people who then enter residential care there is an increase in this onset, which can perhaps be partly explained by a lack of focus on appropriate needs and wants (Sayce, 2000). As carers, either professional or non-professional, there is a need to ask why these rates are so high and how we can identify people suffering or at risk of suffering from yet another problem. The implications of how we identify the person's needs and wishes are vital to how we consequently support them.

Societal views of dementia

To understand an individual's perspective we first need to understand our own values and attitudes and we must consider the implications of how we view people with dementia and consequently label them. Over many years the transformation of how we look at people with mental health problems, including those with dementia, has changed considerably.

The recognition that mental ill health is an illness in the 19th century meant that people were considered to be in need of help or restraint rather than burning at the stake for witchcraft. During the 19th and 20th centuries the professionals took over control of madness, and people with dementia were part of that system. This involved moving people into institutions and the introduction of mental health law to protect the public and the patient. During this time there were many interesting therapies on offer, such as moral therapy. This emphasised strengthening patients' self-control and creating calming environments which induced controlled activity. Much of the use of moral therapy meant that patients had to be confined in institutions and were labelled a danger to society. The introduction of the Mental Treatment Act in 1930 meant that anyone deemed to meet the criteria of mental illness and therefore considered a danger to society could be taken into and kept in hospital indefinitely.

Many attempts to improve the lot of the community by protecting it from the mentally ill have seen a progression on developments in how our society deals with it. The moral therapy of the early 1900s gave way to the mental hygiene movement, and then to control and restraint in the 1970s and 1980s, which all continued to require the use of institutions for control of these people (Sayce, 2000).

During the 1990s things began to change, with the use of more empowering approaches. The Brain Disease Model explained that mental illness should be seen as a disease of the brain which is no different from the disease of any other organ in the body. This theory expelled the idea that mental illness was a moral weakness, or the fault of parents or the environment. However, it meant that there was no responsibility for actions taken by the patients, thus removing their right to make their own decisions about anything. This approach also ignored the fact that there is much evidence to suggest that poverty and environment have a significant effect on rates of illness. Ultimately, this model puts the professionals in control of the individual in all aspects of the patient's life. This meant that anyone suffering from dementia would automatically be taken into a care setting and all the decisions concerning their daily lives would be made for them. Whilst this may seem like a safe and caring option, it means that not only is the person coping with the emotional trauma of dementia, but also with the loss of their free will and self-determination, which all go to make up the individual.

An alternative theory to this was the Individual Growth Model, which was effectively a means of measuring emotional well-being, including the capacity to learn, achieve autonomy, be self-aware, enjoy relationships and meet challenges, at one end of a continuum, to ill health at the other end. The theory contends that as people within society we are all on this line somewhere and constantly move up and down it. This offers meaning to symptoms and allows us to view mental illness as part of normal life. Individuals can be seen as people with views, ideas etc., rather than unwell and unable to make any decisions. For example: a person with dementia may become very upset at the dinner table and begin to cry or shout or wander around. Using the brain disease model it would be easy to assume that the illness is causing them to behave in this way and then try to control that by comforting or medicating. However, within the Individual Growth Model approach we can consider why the person is behaving in this way by trying to establish what exactly is upsetting them – for example, food they don't like or a fellow patient they are not comfortable with. Techniques in controlling behaviours and in identifying why will be explored in later chapters. One of the problems with this theory is that the person can be faced with feelings of guilt at causing the problems if they are asked to examine why they are doing it, and this in itself can present negative reactions and consequences.

The more recent introduction of people into community care facilities has led to the rise in nursing homes for older people and those with dementia. This is a direct result of the development of the current emphasis on seeing anyone with mental illness as another member of society who simply needs help to manage their life. The Social Disability Model considers people with any kind of disability as impaired by society rather than by the problem itself. The person with dementia should be able to live in a normal environment with the support they need and therefore live with the problem rather than being seen as a lost soul who needs seclusion and pity. This model means that anyone with dementia could live outside a hospital environment in the same way that someone without dementia could. It does depend on the support services being able to meet all of those needs in the person's home.

However, the assumption of dementia as a disability does neglect the devastating effects of symptoms. Denying the onset of dementia in its severity could add to the fear of what it is or could become, and limit access to services like medications. Szasz (1987), cited in Bowers (1998), claims that mental illnesses are not real and that all illnesses are a physiological malfunction. The use of this idea leads us to question where the behaviours or emotions have come from. If they are not just a result of changes in the brain then what are they?

If we consider a social explanation which says that society creates mental health problems by the conditions it imposes on people, then we begin to compare moral judgements on breaking rules. An example might be the intolerance of bad manners at a dinner table, leading to an aggressive response by fellow diners. The aggression comes from a need to ensure that everyone behaves in a certain way and that no one upsets the equilibrium. Typically, a person with dementia is very vulnerable to these social constraints as they lose the ability to comply with social graces. The consideration of mental health problems being a result of social rule-breaking simply portrays the person with dementia as passive and re-confirms their inability to take responsibility for any decisions in their lives, including something as simple as whether they have their hair brushed at a particular moment in time. A focus on personalising the relationship can be influential in creating a way of communicating and developing rather than simply assuming the deterioration of ability.

The use of these models lies in understanding how society perceives dementia. It helps us to deliberate about the moral dilemmas of care without having to apply the assumption that these factors cause it.

So, what does all this mean? Dementia is a dominant image of old age in our current cultural belief systems (Sayce, 2000), and this means that we often assume it to be normal for people to have dementia when they get old. There are many problems with this assumption:

- Young people also get dementia and have different needs which are often not accounted for, as most of the services are geared to older people.
- If we assume that it is normal to have these problems we will not consider them important and simply control them rather than trying to provide support.
- If dementia is assumed to be a degenerative disease with no positive outlook then the person is sentenced to a slow, painful and depersonalising journey to death.

If, however, we can see the implications of these attitudes and incorporate them into our approach, then we can try to understand just how it feels to have no control of your day-to-day life and, how distressing it is to be unable to recall the names of people who you should know, or understand how much the person needs physical and emotional contact as much as anyone else.

Professional policy and guidelines

The professionals most likely to carry out assessments with people with dementia and their carers are psychiatrists, mental health nurses, social workers, occupational therapists and many other specialist staff within the 'multi-disciplinary team'. The team is made up of all the people who may be needed to help a person and their family in a coordinated and efficient way.

The team are considered to be the specialists who will also be able to offer all the available and up-to-date practical advice and services. They also offer emotional support, and one professional will be appointed to develop a close link with the person and their family so that they are in position of mutual trust during the progression of the problems. The development of this relationship is vital to the smooth running and effective support offered to people. Much research into the need to protect vulnerable people from neglect and abuse has shown that care givers' burden and stress are very influential.

The introduction of the Health Act in 1999 led to a more focused service in which local mental health trust and social care agencies came together with pooled funds, lead commissioning and integrated provision. These three elements of bringing services together can be evaluated as to their effectiveness, but essentially it means that teams are now potentially much more streamlined and efficient. The aim of the legislation was to help the partners of these groups of professionals to design and deliver services around the needs of users, rather than worrying about the limitations of their own organisation's resources – for example, the need for a person to be admitted into or discharged from a hospital ward often brought up practical funding issues, and the NHS and social services staff could often find themselves in a situation where neither had the resource to provide the accommodation needed. This inevitably brought tension within the working relationship. The intention of this new law was to ensure that these professionals were working together with the same priorities and resources and aiming for the same outcome.

Further legislation has come into place since which has attempted to protect users of the services and their carers, and this group of people are often referred to as 'vulnerable people'. The 'No Secrets' guidance (Department of Health, 2000a) is a key document which identifies people who are vulnerable at any age because of illness or disability, and those with dementia are included in this. The need to protect people with dementia is very important, as the incapacitating nature of this problem can lead to good intentions becoming abusive and the attraction of abusers to the individual. This document considered national strategies and the development of the National Service Frameworks in 2000 (for those under 65) and 2001 (for those over 65) made these requirements more specific (Department of Health, 2000b, 2001). These frameworks began to give people with mental health problems and resulting vulnerabilities rights about decisions being made in their interests. Areas particularly relevant to people with dementia were sparse but could be used indirectly. The standards involved mental health promotion, which could be seized upon to promote a positive image of ageing and try to eradicate the assumptions of society that people with dementia are all old and unable to make decisions for themselves. There were attempts to make access to services easier and to provide a more focused assessment of severe illness. The standard identifying the need to care for carers also had great potential and indeed could be seen as a catalyst for the development of further carers' support and its priority. All of the standards in the NSF (under 65) had lots of scope for people with dementia, but little, or no direct relevance. The NSF for older people did improve this a little by leading to the introduction of a national requirement for services to provide a joint approach to assessment. The development of memory clinics was a direct result of this strategy, which now means that anyone with a memory problem will now be seen and assessed in a structured way and considered for current treatments, including new medications.

The proposed framework of assessment considered a clear pathway, as shown in Figure 3.1. This meant that for the first time people with dementia and their carers had a structured and clear pathway of help and support which they could be involved in consistently, simply by being aware of their rights to the service.

The development of legislation continued with the review of the Mental Health Act 1983 which encompasses the introduction of the Human Rights Act 1998 from European law into British Law from 2000. The new legislation is being considered by the Mental Health Commission and is looking at a new perspective on carers' rights, incapacity to consent, Tribunal systems and mental disorder definitions. All of these issues have a profound effect on people with dementia and their carers as they are all aimed at promoting a more empowering and thus informed integration of professionals' and clients' decision-making processes.

The most recent addition to this type of legislation was the passing of the Mental Capacity Act in April 2005. The emphasis of this act is on presumption of capacity, maintaining personal choice and acting in best interests. Although the detail may change before it becomes law in 2007, its principal aim, to empower people through accurate diagnosis of capacity to consent, is potentially a very powerful means of ensuring that people with dementia retain their human rights.

So, although currently assessment of the person with dementia and their carers is ideologically in the best interests of those people, there are issues

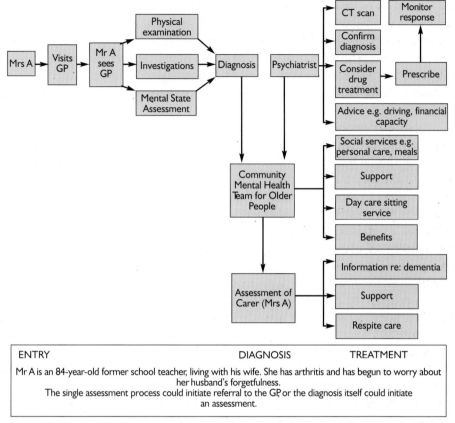

Figure 3.1 Care pathway for dementia (Department of Health, 2001, p. 102; Crown Copyright).

which need to be faced by those of us doing that assessment and caring for them as a result of our conclusions. This expanding legal framework will continue to develop and the care offered must continue with it.

Assessment by health and social care professionals

Most professionals use a structured, although adapted, model of assessment. Some of these have already been mentioned – the Mini Mental State (Folstein *et al.*, 1975), Neuropsychiatric Inventory (Cummings *et al.*, 1994), the Cognitive Profile (Bolland *et al.*, 1996), the Modified Mini-Cog (Borson *et al.*, 2000) and CAMDEX-R (Roth *et al.*, 1998). Further established tools include the Information–Memory–Concentration test (IMC) (Blessed *et al.*, 1968), the Clifton Assessment Procedures (CAPE) (Pattie and Gilleard, 1979), the Cambridge

Cognitive Examination (CAMCOG) (Bolland *et al.*, 1997) and many other tools are used and adapted to the needs of services and their users.

However, one of the problems with these tools is that they are adapted and therefore cannot be used easily to identify national trends and information for research. The need to use data gained from assessments is vital to continuing with the development of quality care, and the individuality of this process often hinders that.

There are also issues with each tool's reliability (retest accuracy) and validity (does it measure what it should?). For example, with tools such as the Mini Mental State examination, the testing relies on a certain educational level, which may hinder the person's performance. This could result in a low score due to a lack of original academic ability and a consequent conclusion of intellectual decline. With tests like this there are also problems when different assessors measure the same client and find that the scores vary. This can often be down to lack of experience, but it essentially means that a person's problems could be rated inaccurately. With the more multi-dimensional tools, such as the CAPE, it is possible for assessors to consider the categories in line with their own culture and be unaware of the social networks or internal resources resulting from belief systems that an individual from another culture might exhibit or prioritise.

The professionals must decide on the most appropriate tool to use within their own service based on key factors:

- National and legal requirements – e.g. use of medication or the provision of memory clinics
- The local population's needs – e.g. cultural and ethnic differences and priorities like adaptation of diet or language resources, age and expectations of society, and social or economic influence on illness
- Individual risk – e.g. considering the needs of each person rather than having a blanket service provision based on assumptions that all old people lose their memory and need to be looked after
- Individual aspirations and hopes for the future – e.g. the wants of an individual rather than just their needs
- Carer relationships – e.g. the combination of, rather than conflict between, the carer and sufferer and professional

The joined-up nature of assessment between professionals means that the approach can be much broader than before, as the team will be assessing the overall impact of the problems of dementia together. However, to ensure that certain information is gathered by the one assessor there needs to be a local strategy for a structured assessment tool. Different professionals will concentrate on their own specialisms once the overall assessment of needs and wants has been established.

Initial interviews should consider aspects of:

- Cognitive deterioration and the effect of this on the sufferer and carer. This may involve the use of some of the measurement tools mentioned previously.
- A baseline measure of capacity to consent at this stage is vital to ensure that the person with dementia has all the appropriate chances to make day-to-day or legal decisions about their future, and also provides a measurement for comparison later.
- Development of an awareness of social structures, networks, needs and likes. This can be based on some relationship and life story history which will offer key information into the potential benefits or problems ahead in this caring relationship. The financial assessment of need can often highlight poverty and neglect through lack of awareness.
- Baseline assessment of mood and psychological states of sufferer and carer. As we know, depression rates are high in people with high care-giver stress and in people with dementia. Overstall (2005) identifies the need to look for signs of depression automatically and consistently, such as: loss or increase in appetite or weight, insomnia or excess sleepiness, retardation or agitation, loss of energy or fatigue, feelings of worthlessness or guilt, impaired concentration and suicidal thoughts. These symptoms must continue over two weeks, occur on most days and cause significant social or functional impairment.
- Establish a baseline of the person's verbal communication skills. This will allow a plan to be made which can be consistently applied by all involved in communicating effectively, whether by use of observations, touch or prompts.
- Identify levels of distress and patterns of behaviour or stimulus for these. For example, the individual may be in pain because of constipation and an imprecise assessment could lead to conclusions that they are generally distressed and need behaviour modification care or medication.
- Establish realistic levels of risk in conjunction with the priorities of the main carer. The lay person's version of what risk is will always differ from the professional's, as a professional will use aggregated risk (e.g. what is likely according to statistics), while the carer will use the specifics of what they see and feel (Shaw and Shaw, 2001). The question of whether assessment can ever be empowering comes back to risk assessment and lies firmly in the ability of the professional body being able to say that some risks are acceptable if balanced against quality of life needs. The use of assistive technology tools may help to improve the need of the health and social care services to rescue everyone from perceived risk.

Assessment by carers

Most carers are not health or social care professionals and yet they have an enormous capacity to adapt their lifestyles and become very skilled at the job. The carer is the first contact that a person with dementia has and is therefore incredibly important in guiding the process of care overall. The essential nature of the relationship will of course depend on the history of the relationship prior to the onset of dementia. For example, for a couple who have had a very loving relationship, the strain of caring for someone who no longer contributes to that can be very distressing, and may even cause feelings of resentment. Consequent changes in the relationship may also engender a feeling of fear or anxiety for the carer and the sufferer if the pair has not really ever understood each other's needs (Carpenter and Dave, 2004). If the relationship prior to the onset of the problems was already problematic then the changes can also bring these feelings to the fore, and they may include anger and frustration.

Current research into the well being of carers is being carried out considering the effect of sufferers' behaviour on carers' ability to cope. Preliminary findings suggest that many carers suffer from depression; many are at risk of jeopardising their own health; almost all carers have coped with similar behavioural and psychological symptoms from the sufferers; and ultimately that there is a relationship between care-giver depression and these behaviours and between care-giver depression and relationship quality (Campbell *et al.*, 2004). Other research identifies the importance of carers' needs being assessed by use of their own descriptions and processes of priority (Bucks *et al.*, 1996). The use of the carer rating scale called the 'Bristol Activities of Daily Living' has helped to enhance accuracy in the assessment, as the professional and carer work together to consider the most important issues in each individual situation. The use of criteria which are prioritised by the full-time carer means that the assessment is much more balanced and focused on sufferer and carer alike.

Practical aspects of a home assessment:

- Ask your health professional, nurse/social worker/doctor what kind of things you need to look out for
- Access legal information from organisations such as the Alzheimer's Society, MIND and Age Concern. The protection of a vulnerable person is a vital part of shielding the person and the carer from different types of problem, such as abuse or loss of rights. Professionals can offer up to date information on the appropriate use of financial and human rights protection frameworks, such as power of attorney, enduring power of attorney and court of protection.
- Spend time recording significant events. A daily diary is not necessary, as this would become very time-consuming and potentially tiresome. Record-

ing key behaviours, responses and feelings at times of day may help to identify developing problems or patterns of existing ones.

- Read about dementia and its problems and consider the need for some peer
  support by contacting local voluntary agencies like the Alzheimer's Society
  or MIND.
- Spend time with the person you are caring for, trying to communicate in
  whatever way is possible. This will help you to re-establish a connection
  with them, if it has been lost, by simply recognising each other on a regular basis. This can be for short periods of time, but significant in its content, and can be as simple as holding hands. The time you spend can offer
  you valuable insight into what each of you needs to calm down difficult
  situations as well as how to develop the relationship you may be grieving
  for.
- Monitor and try to record physical ability, like eating, walking and talking,
  so that you have a measure of improvement or decline. This will help you to
  work with the professionals in getting practical support like feeding aids or
  mobility appliances.
- Consider the reasons for any mood changes or aggressive/hostile behaviours. There is usually a reason for changes in behaviour or mood which can
  be traced back to the environment or people around the person with dementia. This can be things like new routines, changes in wallpaper, responses to
  medication, hallucinations, hostility from carers, general boredom or frustration at the person's own inabilities. If you can understand the problem
  then you will be able to deal with it more effectively.

The remaining chapters will concentrate on offering help and guidance to
people who have dementia and those who care for them. The results of interviews with people in this situation have structured the approach. The issues
identified as areas of concern or need are those highlighted by these people.
Each chapter will be focused on the key issues, and will be put into context by
a short introduction of quotes from the interview respondents.

The group were kind enough to volunteer their time to discuss a very significant and potentially painful part of their lives with the author, and for this we
offer sincere thanks. The Alzheimer's Society approached a number of people
in a local area in one region of England. This means that the comments are not
going to represent the whole of the British community. This, however, is seen
as acceptable by the author, as this is a not a research project and the outcome
is not to prove a point, but simply to ensure that the principle of this book (i.e. a
person-focused approach) is adhered to and that those talked about make valuable contributions.

Despite this, it is clear that ethnic differences, sexual identity issues, homeless people or those outside of the services are not considered within this focus.
This can be an area for development and evaluation of service inclusion.

References

Blessed, G., Tomlinson, B. E. and Roth, M. (1968) The association between quantitative measures of dementia and of senile change in the cerebral grey matter of elderly subjects. *British Journal of Psychiatry*, **114**, 797–811.

Borson, S., Scanlan, J., Brush, M., Vitaliano, P. and Dokmak, A. (2000) The Mini-Cog: a cognitive 'vital signs' measure for dementia screening in multilingual elderly. *International Journal of Geriatric Psychiatry*, **15**, 1021–7.

Bolland, G., Buckley, C., Bucks, R., Emmerson, C., Hooper, J. and McManus, M. (1996) *The Cognitive Profile (Cog-Pro): a Practical Approach to Cognitive Assessment of Older Adults*. Dementia Voice Publications, Bristol.

Bowers, L. (1998) *The Social Nature of Mental Illness*. Routledge, London.

Bucks, R. S., Ashworth, D. L., Wilcock, G. K. and Siegfried, K. (1996) Assessment of activities of daily living in dementia: development of the Bristol Activities of Daily Living scale. *Age and Ageing*, **25**, 113–20.

Campbell, P., Jones, L., Bentham, P. and Lendon, C. (2004) An investigation of the impact of behavioural and psychological symptoms of dementia on carer well being. *9th International Conference on Dementia*. Alzheimer's Society, Philadelphia.

Carpenter, B. and Dave, J. (2004) Patient–spouse concordance in health care and psychosocial preferences. *9th International Conference on Dementia*. Alzheimer's Society, Philadelphia.

Cummings, J., Mega, M., Gray, K., Rosenberg-Thompson, S., Carusi, D. A. and Gornbein, J. (1994) The Neuropsychiatric Inventory: comprehensive assessment in dementia. *Neurology*, **44**, 2308–14.

Department of Heath (2000a) *No Secrets: Guidance on Developing and Implementing Multi-agency Policies and Procedures to Protect Vulnerable Adults From Abuse*. HMSO, London.

Department of Heath (2000b) *National Service Framework for Mental Health*. HMSO, London.

Department of Health (2001) *National Service Framework for Older People*. HMSO, London

Folstein, M., Folstein, S. and McHugh, P. (1975) 'Mini-mental state'. A practical method for grading the cognitive state of patients for the clinician. *Journal of Psychiatric Research*, **12**, 189–98.

Norman, I. and Redfern, S. (1997) *Mental Health Care for Elderly People*. Churchill Livingstone, Edinburgh.

Office for National Statistics (2000) *Psychiatric Morbidity among Adults Living in Private Households, 2000*. http://www.statistics.gov.uk/downloads/theme_health/psychmorb.pdf.

Overstall, P. (2005) How to recognise depression in dementia. *Journal of Dementia Care*, **13**(3), 24-26.

Pattie, A. H. and Gilleard, C. J. (1979) *Manual of Clifton Assessment Procedures for the Elderly (CAPE)*. Hodder & Stoughton Educational, Sevenoaks.

Roth, M., Huppert, F., Mountjoy, C. and Tym, E. (1998) *CAMDEX-R: The Cambridge Examination for Mental Disorders of the Elderly*, 2nd edn. Cambridge University Press, Cambridge.

Sayce, L. (2000) *From Psychiatric Patient to Citizen – Overcoming Discrimination and Social Exclusion*. Macmillan Press, London.

Shaw, A. and Shaw, I. (2001) Risk research in a risk society. *Research Policy and Planning*, **19**(1), 3–16.

CHAPTER 4

The process of interviewing and finding out what people want and need

Learning points on legal and ethical aspects of developing care:

■ Gaining individual perspective and the importance of this information to develop care strategies
■ Legal and political influence on care practice
■ Quality of life care development
■ The research input of this text and its ethical concerns
■ The interviews transcribed and explained

Accessing the individual perspective

The decision to make this book focus on the issues identified by those concerned was one of ethical, practical and legal consideration. The need to ensure that people's lives are represented realistically needed to be weighed against the need to protect vulnerable people and maintain their right to protection.

Legal, political and professional influence

The emphasis now on person-centred care is justified by the very nature of its action, which is to ensure client independence and control of their own lives. However, the very nature of this debate does mean that carers, especially professionals, have to balance the needs of the vulnerable and their safety with their basic human rights.

The need for empowerment is strong within the statutory services, working in balance with protecting people from harm. Many recent and current Government strategies have centred on this issue and can be seen as moving the care role forward. This move takes care into a new era of being client-focused and taking acceptable risks from the old style of service-oriented care which attempts to eradicate risk altogether. Many people feel that the need to eliminate risk is paramount, but the situation is more complex than whether carers protect people or not – it concerns quality of life and the individual's right to make decisions. Whilst this may lead to taking greater risks, it does provide a means by which people can continue to live as independently and potentially contentedly as possible.

Relevant policies and guidance offered by the Government and other support organisations help to clarify the current move in this way.

As a result of *The New NHS: Modern, Dependable* (Department of Health, 1997), frameworks for care standards were identified for numerous areas of illness and care. This included one for mental health and one for older people. *The National Service Framework for Mental Health* (Department of Health, 2000a) and *The National Service Framework for Older People* (Department of Health, 2001b) have been the two documents which can be most useful to people with dementia and their carers. It is as a result of the latter document that memory clinics were established, thus ensuring that anyone suspected of having dementia would be assessed, using the same standards across the country, for care needs and medication.

Further documents have considered the needs of those with dementia more closely, and the current evaluation of the Mental Health Act 1983 is in the process of debating the need for greater carer influence. The decisions made for those deemed to have lost capacity to consent or make their own decisions is an ethical issue of great proportions, and the integration of the Human Rights Act 1998 into British law has indeed made the argument much more complex. Despite these political concerns the issue does come back to client empowerment versus client safety, and the need for a balance. How we ensure protection for vulnerable people without sacrificing individuality and quality of life is the debate.

The *Forget Me Not* (2000, 2002) documents considered the necessities of remembering the needs of individuals and prioritising client and carer needs over service provision. The changes in care priorities were around seeing a person as an individual rather than seeing a group of people who have dementia and have therefore lost any human rights for dignity and compassion in their time of need. Vulnerable adults include any person who depends on others for their care through illness, disability etc., and people with dementia come under this umbrella. This group were to be provided with some kind of safety standard through *No Secrets* (Department of Health, 1999), which identified a need to acknowledge vulnerabilities and actively protect people from harm by abuse or neglect.

These organisations offer guidance and research based strategies to enhance the Department of Health policy making and provide individuals with support.

- The Alzheimer's Society: http://www.alzheimers.org.uk/
- CJD Support Network: http://www.cjdsupport.net/
- MIND: http://www.mind.org.uk/
- Carers UK: http://www.carersuk.org/
- Age Concern: http://www.ageconcern.org.uk/
- Huntington's Disease Association: http://www.hda.org.uk/

An example of this combined approach to providing services can be found in the latest edition of *Who Cares: Information and Support for Carers of People with Dementia* (Department of Health, 2004b). This document was originally devised in 2000 and consists of information about dementia, daily lives and help available. It was resourced and written by the Alzheimer's Society, Help the Aged, Age Concern, The Princess Royal Trust for Carers, Dementia Voice and the South London and Maudsley NHS Trust.

Alzheimer's Disease International (2000) has also produced a 'Charter of principles' which offers some guidance to carers and people with dementia on the rights of that individual:

- Alzheimer's Disease and related dementias are progressive, incapacitating diseases of the brain that have a profound effect on persons with dementia and members of their families.
- A person with dementia continues to be a person of worth and dignity, and deserving of the same respect as any other human being.
- People with dementia need a physically safe living environment and protection from exploitation and abuse of person and property.
- People with dementia require information and access to coordinated medical and welfare services. Anyone who is thought to have the disease needs medical assessment and those with the disease require ongoing care and treatment.
- People with dementia should as far as possible participate in decisions affecting their daily lives and future care.
- The family carers of a person with dementia should have their needs relating to the care assessed and provided for and should be enabled to take an active role in the process.
- Adequate resources should be available and promoted to support people with dementia and their carers throughout the course of the disease.
- Information, education and training on the disease, its effects and how to provide care must be available to all those involved in the assistance of people with dementia.

Another aspect of change of direction has been in the combination approach of services. The Health and Social Care Act 2001 stipulates the need for collaborative care and education. This includes the involvement of service users and their carers, educationalists and professionals. It builds on the aims of integrating health and local authority services for vulnerable people. This means that the service should be much more focused, and less repetitive and counterproductive. New care trusts were set up which could commission and provide services which combine the professional care and services of health and social care. There have been many issues with this strategy, including which partner is dominant and services being charged financially for not achieving combined objectives. Despite this, the strategy takes the whole care agenda into a different and potentially useful new phase of client-centred rather than service-centred care approaches. The *Independence, Wellbeing and Choice* (Department of Health, 2005b) Green Paper is being debated in government at the time of writing and is developing this theme in more detail by emphasising the shared service provision as integral to successful promotion of person centred care for all.

Supporting People with Long Term Conditions (Department of Health, 2005a) is a model for NHS and social care professionals to use when setting up new services or reviewing existing arrangements. This document is based on the premise that vulnerable people rarely have only one problem, and this model of strategic care may help services to ensure that people get all the help they need without any aspects being neglected. The document assumes that unnecessary use of emergency care and therefore inefficient financial management have led to poor use of resources. The claim is that this strategy will have the effect of ensuring that community care is a priority, and this will be demonstrated by a reduction in the use of inpatient emergency bed days of 5% by 2008.

The Carers (Equal Opportunities) Act (Department of Health, 2004a) means that all carers have a legal framework of rights from which to ensure they are part of the process of decision making in any care planning.

The Care Standards Act (Department of Health, 2000c) set out the requirements for people being placed in care settings to ensure assessments are equitable throughout the country. This was closely followed by *Care Homes for Older People: National Minimum Standards* (Department of Health, 2001a) which set out to standardise and regulate the care offered when people are placed in a care home.

Many new strategies have been put in place for educational and workforce change which address the issue of using each other's expert knowledge to enhance our combined development and ultimately the individual's quality of life.

The last aspect of change involves the introduction of the 'capacity to consent' into a legal framework in the Mental Capacity Act 2005. Although there have always been standards for assessing whether individuals have the capacity to make decisions about their life depending on their mental state, there is a movement to ensure that people who have lost that ability during illness or disability like dementia are protected. The human rights of these individuals are paramount, and the Act begins by assuming that everyone has capacity to make a decision about their own life until proven otherwise. This means that a diagnosis of dementia or any other debilitating problem does not automatically mean the removal of decision-making rights. The Act talks about many aspects of big life decisions like finance and care plans, but this issue is larger than that. These require the person with dementia and the carer to consider which decisions they can and cannot still take despite the problems of forgetting and loss of ability to rationalise or comprehend. The assumption of incapacity is especially dangerous when we look at day-to-day activities such as whether or not a person wants to eat a particular item of food and the right of that individual to refuse. Current cultures of care often tend towards the assumption that people with dementia can and will eat whatever they are given and that this is not even a choice which should be offered. In defence of many carers and services, this is not the case, but it serves as an example. The choice of which food to eat not being given to the person can lead to them becoming frustrated and hostile, leading the carer to assume they don't want to eat rather than the idea that they just don't want to eat this particular food. As will be discussed in later chapters, consent is not only about the big life-changing decisions, it comes back to basic self-determination and affects simple life tasks.

The individual perspective

As a result of this change in care culture, the emphasis of this book is to ensure that its content is relevant to people with dementia, carers and professionals. To do this, it was necessary to identify the issues that come up for these groups in everyday life and to consider their responses in coping with them.

The process of getting the information took the form of approaching the Alzheimer's Society in Mansfield, Nottinghamshire, and discussing the plan and reasoning behind the book. The team there were extremely helpful and they spent time explaining the request to users of their service and asking them if they would like to take part.

It was always assumed that any person who agreed to participate could withdraw at any stage, including after the interview. The information given could be withdrawn up until the point of going to publishers, and respondents were given contact details to do so (Appendix 2). As a direct result of this link the interviews took place with 10 pairs of carers and sufferers. The pairings included mainly wives and husbands, but there were a few mother and daughter contributions. Each interview had the same format, and was recorded and then transcribed into the text verbatim. This means that all the comments made by the respondents are in context and therefore understandable and not misleading (Appendix 1).

This required consideration of capacity to consent and whether people with dementia should be asked to contribute information, as they might not be able to give consent. Indeed, one woman who was interviewed has dementia and gave her consent, but it was felt by the author that her capacity to consent was limited, as she could not recall clearly what she was consenting to. Therefore her data was not used. The other people with dementia were represented by their carers and any comments they made were made in conjunction with the carer, and it is assumed for the purposes of this work that a combined consent is appropriate, as each respondent could support the other. Despite this, there are still some concerns about the nature of consent by the people with dementia and the extent of their ability to agree to information being given out about them in this form. The author acknowledges the need for further evidence of consent, but this work is about valuing contributions, and is in no way to benefit others deceitfully or to cause harm intentionally or unintentionally. The individuals interviewed all gave consent at the time and agreed to the nature of the questions. They also agreed to the format and the publication of their comments, thus indicating approval of the process at the time of questioning. All were able to comprehend the issues, and the comments of those who could not are not used.

In this vein, each interview started with an explanation of the book and its purpose. Also emphasised was the right to withdraw at any time up until the text went to the publisher, and the implications of discussing such issues with a stranger. Thankfully, all the respondents were keen to tell their stories, and any signs of distress led to the interview being put on hold with an option of stopping, and counselling taking place. All the respondents were asked if they would like to be anonymous, and they chose whether or not to use their own names. They were informed of the issue of being identifiable via the geographical area and made an informed decision about this. Despite this, to protect sufferers further, the names of the carers who gave consent are the only ones used. Sufferers, friends and professionals are not named at all.

As can be seen in the interview transcripts, the themes are common and yet diverse, and they offer the reader an insight into the workings of life with dementia by those living it.

In the other chapters the comments are broken up into themes for development, but this chapter simply shows the raw feeling, practicalities and general issues faced by these people.

References

Alzheimer's Disease international (2000) *World Alzheimer's Day Bulletin.* Alzheimer's Disease International, London.

Audit Commission (2000, 2002) *Forget Me Not.* http://www.audit-commission.gov.uk/.

Bluglass, R. and Rawnsley, K. A. (1981) *Guide to the Mental Health Act.* Churchill-Livingstone, London.

Dimond, B. and Barker, F. (1999) *Mental Health Law for Nurses.* Blackwell Science, London.

Department of Health (1983) *Mental Health Act (England/Wales).* HMSO, London.

Department of Health (1993) *Code of Practice to the Mental Health Act 1983.* HMSO, London.

Department of Health (1995) *Mental Health Act (Patients in the Community).* HMSO, London.

Department of Health (1997) *The New NHS: Modern, Dependable.* HMSO, London.

Department of Health (1999) *No Secrets: The Protection of Vulnerable Adults.* HMSO, London.

Department of Health (2000a) *Reforming the Mental Health Act, Summary.* HMSO, London.

Department of Health (2000b) *Care Standards Act.* HMSO, London.

Department of Health (2000c) *The National Service Framework·for Mental · Health.* HMSO, London.

Department of Health (2001a) *Care Homes for Older People: National Minimum Standards.* HMSO, London.

Department of Health (2001b) *The National Service Framework for Older People.* HMSO, London.

Department of Health (2004a) *Carers (Equal Opportunities) Act.* HMSO, London.

Department of Health (2004b) *Who Cares? Information and Support for the Carers of People with Dementia.* HMSO, London.

Department of Health (2005a) *Supporting People with Long Term Conditions: an NHS and Social Care Model to Support Local Innovation and Integration.* HMSO, London.

Department of Health (2005b) *Independence, Well-Being and Choice: Our Vision for the Future of Social Care for Adults in England.* HMSO, London.

Jones, R. (2000) *Mental Health Act Manual*, 6th edn. Sweet and Maxwell, London.

McCreadie, C. (1998) Elder abuse: issues for nurses. *Nursing Times*, **94**(45), 60–1.

Mental Capacity Act (2005) http://www.opsi.gov.uk/acts/acts2005/20050009.htm.

Northcote, N., Charity, K. and Neal, K. (2000) What do you do when your sense of right is challenged by those in authority? *Nursing Times*, **96**(16), 31.

Parker, C. (2001) Briefing: The Human Rights Act 1998. *Mental Health Care and Learning Disabilities*, **4**(5), 174–5.

Pedlar, M. (1999) *MIND the Law*. MIND Publications, London.

Penhale, B. and Kingston, P. (1997) Elder abuse: the role of risk management. *British Journal of Community Health Nursing*, **2**(4), 201–6.

Pitkeathley, J. (1994) Carers' perspectives. *Nursing Times*, **3**(22), 1171–2, 1189–90.

Quigley, L. (2000) Screen test. *Community Care*, 16 March, 26–7.

Slater, P. and Eastman, M. (1999) *Elder Abuse: Critical Issues in Policy and Practice*. Age Concern, England.

Tomlin, S. (1992) *Abuse of the Elderly: an Unnecessary and Preventable Problem*. British Geriatric Society, London.

Wertheimer, A. (1993) *Speaking Out: Citizen Advocacy and Older People*. Centre for Policy on Ageing, London.

The interview transcripts

All the questions came from a number of main themes, which were of a standard based on the interviewer;s research and experience of what information was needed. The questions had a semi-structured format leading off from the themes and were guided very much by the experience and insight offered by the expertise of the person with dementia and their carers. The combination of the three different perspectives directing the interviews meant that appropriate, relevant and useful information can be used from these interviews and individuals.

Each theme and its main direction is explained here.

Theme 1: The feelings associated with dementia entering a person's life

This theme and question were devised to try to encourage respondents to explore the feelings they had about the problems. A more practically based question would not invite them to describe their feelings. So, despite the risk of the persons discussing upsetting issues, it was more important to encourage this expression and then ensure that the consenting adult was able to convey the true extent of how they felt. Any distress was acknowledged at the time and no one felt pressured to continue if upset. All respondents were interviewed with empathy and compassion and not left alone with upsetting feelings having been surfaced.

Q: How did you feel when you found out you had dementia?

I cried a lot. I thought they were going to come and take me away. I didn't think anything was wrong (*D. Levers*)

Can't remember that (*Anon 2*)

He was told and he was saying that's it, I'm going to die. I assumed he didn't remember later as we never talked about it (*W. Booth*)

I thought I was going daft, I didn't like that but got used to it and you learn to live with it (*B. Hargreaves*)

Mum got really defensive when asked assessment questions 'cause she didn't know the answers (*B. Butcher*)

Q: How do you feel about the problems you are having with your memory?

I thought it was getting worse... Memory gradually coming over... I was doing things that I couldn't do (*S. Hubbert*)

I wasn't as quick as I should have been, couldn't remember (*B. Hargreaves*)

Q: How did you feel when the person was diagnosed with dementia and you were to become a carer?

Couldn't take it in at first (*M. Hubbert*)

I couldn't really believe it at first, felt like it was happening to someone else. It was quite a shock. All these years she's been looking after me, now we have to look after each other (*P. Levers*)

He went to Millbrook, I knew there was something with his memory. When they told what was wrong I was quite shocked, and I kept it to myself. I didn't want to admit what was wrong. Took me a while to accept it, still thought it was his age until things got a bit worse (*Anon 1*)

Nigel is 47 years old. He fell ill three years before diagnosis. Initially we were told that he didn't have it. Then one afternoon the nurse told me that it was positive. It was devastating 'cause we really thought he hadn't got it, I was on my own. Previously we thought it may be dementia because his Dad and uncle both died from it in 40–50 years old. I felt devastated; how would we cope as I am disabled too? But obviously we had to. Because we couldn't talk about I got frustrated and we used to fight all the time. He just shut himself away. I talked about it to my CPN and A Society, they were very good (*W. Booth*)

I couldn't take it in at first (*L. Hargreaves*)

When she can't do things she gets frustrated (*Linda H., daughter*)

She was 55 when it started and we really thought it was depression. She cried when I said she should see a doctor. She felt it was me getting on at her. I said I would leave her if she wouldn't go to the doctor, so she agreed. It all started to get so as I was drinking whisky every night as they were so slow in doing anything.

Make sure you are passed on to the specialists as quickly as possible and get the help you will need (*B. Taylor*)

Numb, surprised, emotional, not wanting to face the truth. He said he had Alzheimer's but Alf didn't really understand. We came from the hospital trying to let it soak in and think about what might happen. You think what we will do now. We tried to forget about it but couldn't.. He was 67 years old. Once he knew what it was he got so that he needed looking after (*B. Taylor*)

I wasn't surprised; he was acting strangely for a long time. There were things going on and the GP sent him Millbrook MH Unit and diagnosed straight away. I knew it would be dementia and I felt some relief that it wasn't my imagination. My husband had no recognition of it at all. He asked once what is Alzheimer's but doesn't understand (*Mrs Carr*)

I didn't realise what it meant until I thought about more. I didn't know anything about it and then as things begin to happen more you get to know more about it. (*B. Butcher*)

I saw the woman from Alzheimer's Society and remember telling her I felt that my life was over, I had no life of my own any more. All I had to do was the caring. I thought I was prepared but I wasn't. I had to learn to live with it. Problems had been going on for about 18 months before we went to the doctor. Someone said to us she should be assessed, we felt there was no need and she was just being awkward. A few months later and it all just kept happening, and we decided it wasn't right and so we went to the doctors. She was referred for an assessment. This was delayed because we were in a different catchment area to the doctor from where her address was. Then quickly, someone came and assessed her at home. Then they said it was Alzheimer's (*B. Butcher*)

Q: What were the early symptoms?

First of all she got epileptic, fell and hit her head. That was about 12 years ago. It's all been coming on about 12 years, dementia.

Forgetting people time and places really, not much at the beginning, it just gradually got worse (*M. Hubbert*)

We knew there was something wrong about year before. Started to come back from shops not able to remember names of people she met. Just forgetting things and it started to get worse. She was very depressed and the anti-depressant helped (*P. Levers*)

We went out with one of the grandchildren one day and he was really sharp with them, and it upset me (*Anon 1*)

Losing his keys, unable to sleep, to cope with life in general, initially put it down to stress and anxiety and depression and OCD. He had those symptoms (*W. Booth*)

At the early stages he could still rationalise and make big decisions (*W. Booth*)

Forgetting was the first and I didn't go out much (*B. Hargreaves*)

I thought it was depression at first 'cause her Mum had just died. We had always been really close and then she stared caring less and less about me. I thought we were just growing apart. She would get confused about our usual stuff and she forgot things. Gave a woman in the shop her purse to take the money out. She didn't remember I was sick one time. She stopped doing the shopping properly. Her driving got erratic. All before the diagnosis. When it was all happening I was lost, bewildered and angry. Maureen did everything and I didn't know how to do anything – cook, shop or anything. Everything was blown apart. I was really angry with everybody and expected professionals to be honest and tell us the truth and do what they say they will. She got upset 'cause she wanted to carry on doing things and was aware that she couldn't (*G. Platt*)

We tried to forget but couldn't 'cause of the misunderstandings. Like he was meant to meet me and didn't, he was at home and had completely forgotten. I just didn't say anything. Another time we went on hols and on the way back he got completely lost when driving home. He got so frustrated and angry. I could remember some of it but had to let him do it because he was so upset. His mood was nice at times and other times he got so frustrated 'cause he didn't know what was going on and he was frustrated with every-one, not like him. He said it was getting too much for him, then he would forget about until something else happened (B. Taylor)

When on hols he left my things on the beach and lost all responsibility for his actions. This was different to how he was before. He started saying he couldn't keep up at work, his colleagues at work were phoning me and tell-ing me he wasn't coping. Fortunately he retired around that time anyway. He has a love of music and he used to make sound tapes for shows and things and then he just couldn't do it. He stopped being interested in the house. Things needed doing and he just wouldn't do it. His personal care started to deteriorate. I had to tell him to shave or put on a clean shirt or wash. I just started to feel he wasn't my husband and not the man I married, he was not a man I liked any more (Mrs Carr)

Q: What were the early problems?

She didn't really get lost, a few times wandered away in town but not far. Doesn't leave the house without me (M. Hubbert)

He told me once before he was diagnosed that he couldn't tell the time. Apart from that it was mainly just forgetting. He was still dressing, wash-ing, driving. I knew the driving was not as good 'cause if we were going to my son's he would go to my daughter's. When we were on hols he went to toilet block and got lost for two hours. It was very gradual. He was not depressed about it, neither of us were, we just accepted it 'cause he wasn't too bad. As it's progressed things have got worse for us both (Anon 1)

Because I had to do everything he was unable to do anything, I was tired and we ended up arguing a lot (W. Booth)

She was very depressed and they put her on tablets which worked well and she is still on them (L. Hargreaves)

I was very depressed and cried a lot. I feel better now (B. Hargreaves)

Then she started getting really hostile and was very clingy. Started accusing people of doing things to her. She started reminiscing with a friend and sister and this seemed to upset her. She started to hallucinate. She started thinking she was in her Dad's house and trying to throw me out. She was incontinent and wouldn't wear a pad. She got really hostile and wouldn't do anything. She was admitted to hospital for assessment. She was really not looked after and we brought her home against medical advice (G. Platt)

He would try to go out at night saying he wanted out go home; usually I could talk him out of it. He would go out during the day on his own and I persuaded him to wear an identity bracelet. We could still go out but it was difficult, he wandered off a lot. It came in stages, one thing would die down then another thing would start. He always made me tea, then that turned into a cup of water, so I just had to learn to leave him to it and make my own tea. He would be putting the water in all the tea bags and stuff. One evening he put out a cup of vinegar for my son. He would leave the gas on. We started to not be able to leave him alone. He was getting obsessive. His character before was that he was very thorough and this carried on. He was crying a lot and upset, we cried together (*Mrs Taylor*)

Mum did a lot of wandering about, when she was still at home on her own, and on one occasion the police came and she had nearly been run over on the new bypass. People used to bring her home and then phone me 'cause I left my number in the house. It was happening more often. She wasn't eating and lost loads of weight, said she was, and all the shopping was still in the fridge. She went to a local café but at the wrong times. She wasn't washing or dressing properly. We fell out a lot because I didn't know then, and I'd leave her clean stuff out but she didn't put them on or dry herself with toilet paper. She was a very active person before, holidaying on her own after Dad died, so she wanted to continue and I stopped her. This meant we fell out a lot 'cause I was telling her what to do, she felt. The police said it was really serious so I packed her up and took her to my house and she stayed there (*B. Butcher*)

I had just given up work and I tried to work part time but it didn't work and then I found out about Carer's Allowance, so I considered this as a job (*B. Butcher*)

Q: How did you tell other people and how did they react?

We went to see the GP about six years after it started and he sent her to Millbrook (mental health unit) (*M. Hubbert*)

To be honest I didn't tell anyone at first, then I let them guess themselves (*M. Hubbert*)

Went to GP and then we were sent to Kings Mill within a few weeks. We told family but they knew something was wrong (*P. Levers*)

I didn't tell a soul at first. Told them after he showed sharp manner to grand-kids. I went to GP and told him he was forgetting. Nothing wrong; went for brain scan six months later after it got worse. Then we went to Millbrook and had meeting with professionals. Got DLA and help to apply (*Anon 1*)

I was better at explaining it to other people than accepting it myself. I was happy to tell people but I wasn't accepting it. I told as we went along. Didn't feel I had to hide it. His mother couldn't get her head around it and never really accepted it. Other family didn't seem to understand and they avoided it. Friends and neighbours helped a lot (*W. Booth*)

We told family and others so they would understand and not get upset. But they didn't all understand and some will not talk to us (*L. Hargreaves*)

When you look at my mum she looks well and you can't tell, but they don't know how it is (*Linda, daughter*)

I was telling my son about it. I didn't tell people outside of the family really, except a few friends. They all said I should get her a doctor (*G. Platt*)

I just told them and that explained to them his odd behaviour. Everyone was fine, although my son found it hard to accept. Both my son and daughter understand the implications of the illness (*Mrs Carr*)

I told everyone, and everyone was fine (*B. Butcher*)

Q: How did you access help and did it help?

We go to the memory clinic every six months. We don't need any help. We had an assessment and were to get a hand rail on the stairs but it didn't fit. Got a seat for the bath, which helps. I just went down to the Alzheimer's society myself, we go to a monthly support meeting with them. That gives us people who have same problems to talk to. We are just waiting for people from Age Concern to come about finances (*M. Hubbert*)

Got a CPN and went to support group. They told us about Alzheimer's Society (*Anon 1*)

Went to GP and they did tests and scans but never found anything. A neurologist said they he had a 50% chance due to family history, as we knew, but couldn't confirm. Millbrook said the same, the disease wasn't diagnosed as it hadn't progressed (*W. Booth*)

Went to GP six years ago and he sent us to Millbrook very quickly and she was assessed. No other help then (*L. Hargreaves*)

Somebody else put us on to Alzheimer's Society and they are a great help (*Linda, daughter*)

I think Nigel's mother told me about Alzheimer's Society (*W. Booth*)

We went to GP and she had lost weight to 6st 13lbs. When she went to get the diagnosis from a neurologist he was shouting at her for not following his instructions. He just told us it was Alzheimer's, Maureen started crying and said I am too young. He was very abrasive. He prescribed Aricept and got a private prescription. He did put us in touch with Alzheimer's Society. She got Maureen referred to consultant psychiatrist. He came very quickly and helped (*G. Platt*)

He went to MIND, we had a sitting service and he had respite two weeks out of the month, but that meant he lost his routine when he got back. It went on for about ten years and then things got too much and I couldn't do it any more. Social services and the doctor assessed him and he went into a nursing home (*B. Taylor*)

He went to a day centre and he enjoyed that so now he goes two days a week, for about the last two years. I picked up a leaflet at the mental health unit about Alzheimer's Society and I use the support group when I can (*Mrs Carr*)

I saw an advert in the local paper for the Alzheimer's Society and contacted them. And she came to see me, they have really helped me and the infor-mation sheets and meetings are very good. I gave the leaflets to people in the family (*B. Butcher*)

After the diagnosis, a CPN started visiting and a social worker assessed and this lasted for a few months. Then she had to come and stay with us. That meant we had to be reassessed because she had moved catchments. She started a day centre and seemed to enjoy it, she told me she had been doing stuff and I had to learn to go along with her 'cause she thought she had done these things. This has been increased as we needed it to four days. The problem is that you don't get enough information, because they don't know I suppose what will happen, but it would really help (*B. Butcher*)

Q: What kind of treatments did you have, did they help and were there any problems with them?

She's on Aricept, for last three years. Don't know if it works 'cause we don't know how she would have been without it. No side effects or problems.

She got depressed when it started and she knew something was wrong, she had no treatment for that (*M. Hubbert*)

GP put her on some anti-depressant tablets, side effects meant had to change to a different one. Then later put her on Aricept, doing well on 5 mg; then it was increased to 10 mg and she started with diarrhoea and vomiting; reduced back to 5 and been fine since. Got runny nose from citalopram (*P. Levers*)

Started on Aricept which was good, then that changed to Reminyl. Also Ebixa, and that's not helping – has become a bit nasty – and Amisulpiride started and that's good. He did start to get a bit depressed and was staring at wall. CPN came and they doubled the anti-depressant and that helped (*Anon 1*)

I had to fight for Aricept as they hadn't given him a diagnosis. They gave him it eventually. He was better at thinking and could do things methodically. It made him very tired and then he did not want to do much. He got depressed early on and got meds but he did get worse, and then hallucinations medication led to him being very tired and not functioning. The Aricept was stopped as they felt the meds were not helping him any more. I thought he needed more time on them to see. He was sectioned and I felt I had no choice (*W. Booth*)

He had a mini-stroke and a fit and was admitted into hospital. After coming home we were struggling and the consultant felt that he had to come back into hospital to adjust the medication. After a trip out with me I took him back to the ward. After half an hour they phoned and said he had become very aggressive. I went down and they had him on the floor with five people on him I leant down to touch his head and he was crying and then he was fine. They sectioned him because he wasn't orientated, but I told them he's been like that for over a year. The SW spoke to him and determined he could not make a decision. He was aggressive a few times and bad reactions to all the meds they tried (*W. Booth*)

Got Aricept at first but they changed it to Exelon, I don't think it is as good. Government won't pay for the Aricept. Doctor said after trial she could go back on Aricept if it doesn't suit her. I think she is getting worse (*L. Hargreaves*)

She was started on anti-depressants and her Aricept was reduced. They helped her to calm down a lot. She slept a lot and through the night. It really lifted her spirits. The physical side of our relationship returned. She started a day centre. They involved her in projects and I took her out every day. Later, when she began hallucinating, she went into hospital and they tried all sorts of meds that didn't work. The care was abysmal. We found her in her room with a large bump on her head. She was seriously constipated and they hadn't done anything. They had stopped all her drugs and her mini-mental went down to 13 and then the Aricept was not going to be put back on. She started on respite and this was terrible. She was distressed every time she had to go in. I found her without meds or breakfast one time with dried faeces on her legs. I stopped the respite and made a complaint to the hospital. I was so angry. The response was that they justified it all. I've been offered Newark for respite but it's too far away. She's on Ebixa now and is much better now (*G. Platt*)

He tried Aricept but had terrible side effects and that was stopped. Then he had anti-depressants which helped when he was crying all the time. He also had some to calm him down and to help him sleep, and those worked OK, no side effects (*B. Taylor*)

He started on Aricept and he came back to his old self overnight. He started to take an interest in things again and couldn't be bothered before. However, he has gone back down again. He was depressed and just lay on the couch all day and didn't express his feelings, which is normal for his character. They didn't put him on anti-depressants, but the meds he has for his waterworks are an anti-depressant and that seems to have lifted his mood a bit (*Mrs Carr*)

The doctor refused to give her sleeping tablets. She had something to calm her down at one point but it just made her drowsy and sleepy all the time. I stopped it (*B. Butcher*)

Theme 2: Emotional and practical pressures of care for a person with dementia

This theme was again more about the impact of the identified problems on the person and carers. The practical and emotional mix of information was not only to offer an insight into the daily tasks, but also to recognise the impact of the feelings and the coping strategies used.

Q: How do you cope with the emotional and practical pressures of life with these problems?

Household practicalities

No practical problems, I just do everything. If I go out for a short time I lock the door, but she stays where she is anyway (*M. Hubbert*)

We have really helpful neighbours who take us shopping. She can't cook or anything like that. She couldn't go any further than the street on her own (*P. Levers*)

The carers are 24 hours. We do everything for him. He can't do anything, like feed himself, he tries to help but can't (*W. Booth*)

I do all the cooking and our daughters help with it and the cleaning. She would leave the gas on and stuff (*L. Hargreaves*)

She lost interest in any jobs although I tried to involve her before (*G. Platt*)

He does nothing in the house. He used to do all the fixing and do it yourself and now he just says it doesn't need done (*Mrs Carr*)

Socialising

She stopped reading and embroidery. Picks up newspaper and puts it down again, TV is on but she doesn't really watch it. We go to the pub each weekend, I go to my allotment, she goes to day centre once a week and her friends once a week. We go on bus trips and we go down town (*M. Hubbert*)

Don't do what we used to, but still go out and go on coach trips (*P. Levers*)

Used to go out a lot for meals, but only occasionally now. I have to think ahead. We go with some friends that are in the same position and we go out for walks and stuff. We don't go out like we did and we don't do our camping any more. We go on coach tours now and that's OK and we go with our friends (*Anon 1*)

We haven't really changed. We go down the club on a Saturday night. We go on day trips with Alzheimer's Society and their support group. We go for the shopping and stuff. She can't go on her own (*L. Hargreaves*)

I go to a day centre and I like that, I can have a chat and stuff. They've got time for you. Don't want to go more than once a week (*B. Hargreaves*)

He used to enjoy going to MIND and had a sitting service which he enjoyed but then he became hostile with them and MIND had to stop. We still managed to go out and to friends but I knew when to stop (*B. Taylor*)

We only go shopping now. We used to go out all the time and he was out most nights. He wouldn't cope with any of these things any more. He enjoys the day centre, says he wishes I could come. I try to keep busy by going to the gym and seeing friends. I get emotional support from my daughter. I am spiritual but don't go to church. It helps and I don't see this as a burden but a learning curve. I have applied for a part-time post to give me something interesting to do. We can't go on holiday any more because he wanders off (*Mrs Carr*)

Mum goes to day centre four days now. She is always happy to go and comes back fine. I go out when she is at the day centre. We take her everywhere and that is difficult but you have to learn how to deal with her. She won't eat in a restaurant, but I just have to accept that and not worry. In toilets we are in for ages and I have to keep shouting out to people we won't be long (*B. Butcher*)

Remembering

Can't remember my grandson and brother in law but doesn't see them often (*Anon 1*)

I think she is getting worse lately. Constantly repeating the same questions. And she thinks we are all against her and doing things behind her back. We tell her everything but then she forgets (*Linda, daughter*)

She wonders when her mum is coming down and where her baby is lately. She can't take a message on the phone (*L. Hargreaves*)

I don't always remember. I think I should be able to remember this and it gets to me. I have cried. I think I'm not very clever and it gets me down. If I have to do anything they have to tell me (*B. Hargreaves*)

She never talks about us or my Dad, only her mum and sisters. That upsets me sometimes. She doesn't recognise any of us, won't even answer to being called Mum (*B. Butcher*)

Working

He was working as a porter at the hospital, for 25 years, when he went off sick. Redundancy was threatened so he went back. Then after six months he broke down, couldn't cope with travelling on the bus, getting paranoid about people talking about him. Then I said I wouldn't take him in the car and that was the only way he could go. I knew he had to stop work. The he got early retirement on sick grounds. He didn't want to but accepted that he would have a better quality of life (*W. Booth*)

She started to make mistakes at work and her employers were concerned about her. She stopped work after she broke down in tears and was sent home (*G. Platt*)

Driving

Not driving now, used to drive everywhere (*Anon 1*)

She was told not to drive but she kept on because she wanted to keep her job. She would drive really well before but then she couldn't do manoeuvres and was stopping at junctions too long and stuff (*G. Platt*)

He was driving dangerously and eventually the DVLA refused to renew his license but he carried on until managed to sell his car. Now he complains all the time when I'm driving that I am doing it wrong (*Mrs Carr*)

Self caring

I do everything for her, wash her and cut up food. She tells me when she needs to go to the toilet (*M. Hubbert*)

Sometimes doesn't get to the toilet on time. Seen by the nurse, we had to record when and measure the water, she didn't like that. Now she wears incontinence pants. It's usually if she can't get to a toilet, like when shopping (*P. Levers*)

I don't like that (incontinence) (*D. Levers*)

Neither of us have ever slept very well and that is how it is now (*P. Levers*)

Can't put on tops and fasten buttons on my cardigans. Choose my clothes myself. (*D. Levers*)

Does know when to wash and dress (*P. Levers*)

Sometimes struggles to use toilet properly, needs to be guided (*Anon 1*)

Legs are bad and can't get in and out of bath. SS offered a stool, can't lower him. Got sticky things on floor of bath and two rails on side. Can't dress himself. I choose clothes and help him dress. If in bath will wash but forgets to rinse. Can't make tea or cook. Eats less but usually eats everything, knife and fork becoming a problem (*Anon 1*)

We feed and change him as he is doubly incontinent. He walks about a lot and won't sit down to eat. Eats well and usually takes meds. We give him a lot of space to walk around. He hits things and then calms down. The carer sleeps in the room with him and we usually have the same carers (*Booth*)

I put the washing away and she moves it all when tidying (*Linda, daughter*)

I put out her clothes and she dresses, I go on to the shower and remind her to shower and stuff but she does it herself. She eats and drinks fine. She sleeps all night (*L. Hargreaves*)

I've always liked my food. Tastes haven't changed (*B. Hargreaves*)

I do everything for her, toilet, shower, feed, meds, everything. She lost interest and initiative (*G. Platt*)

I had to leave clothes out for him and hope he put them on. Often he put on the wrong things. We laughed about it and that relieved the frustration a lot of the time. I had to wash him, because he was spending too much time doing it, which was his character anyway. He got really frustrated at not washing himself properly. I had to keep encouraging him to sit at the table, but he ate himself when he was sat down. Often I just let him do the dishes when he wanted to keep him occupied. He got to the stage where he didn't know what the toilet was for. He had bowel problems and then it became really difficult because he began to get irritated by me taking him there. We were very often in a mess. The nurse tried to help with meds but it didn't help other than make him incontinent more (*B. Taylor*)

I have to tell him to shave, wash, shower etc. I put his clothes out for him and he can put them on himself. He is not incontinent. He eats and drinks too much. He's had a meal, then an hour later he is in the kitchen getting himself more food. He's put on a stone and a half in weight over the last six months. He does what I tell him (*Mrs Carr*)

Mum's sleep is very poor, she is up all night and then we can't keep her awake during the day. She won't sit on the toilet and she's doubly incontinent, and this all over the floor. I can't get her to sit down. She used to put faces down the radiators and stuff. She takes inco pads off. I found big inco pants and she keeps them on better. She slipped onto the floor on the Kylie sheets so I buy these nappy-type bed covers. Sometimes she's nasty, and will not put them on. So I spend the night checking on her. She still eats, but recognises the cutlery and needs help. I dress her and she mostly lets me. If she's tired she grumbles but we usually get on with it (*B. Butcher*)

Dealing with feelings/frustrations and the effect on others

She doesn't get angry (*M. Hubbert*)

Feel better now because I can go out, although I can't go on my own. I feel better and we do everything together (*D. Levers*)

Started getting a bit nasty. Don't think tablets helping, change since meds changed. Mood is generally very different. He was always very placid before. It upsets me when he snaps at me. Get support from friends and Alzheimer's Society. Family help but I try not to bother them (*Anon 1*)

We let him wander around and calm down himself. If he is out of routine, tired, wet, there are too many people, doesn't like the dark because of the shadows and hallucinations, in pain or just fed up he gets aggressive. He throws things around and hits things, occasionally people but not so much now. Although if he is hallucinating he may grab and hit (*W. Booth*)

Over the last two weeks gradually his mood has been really good. His speech, understanding and alertness much better. The medical profession are very surprised by this and can't explain it. The only thing that has changed is that we have been giving him nutrition drinks three times a day because of weight loss with all the walking he does. He's not normal, all the way through he has been different in his symptoms and surprised the medics. Just now he will understand if you speak slowly, but at night he gets very tearful, not sure if it's tiredness or fed up (*W. Booth*)

I feel good just now, 'cause he's settled, although I know it won't last for ever (*W. Booth*)

I get upset and frustrated when I can't see what I have to do next and I have to ask them. They're very good and they help me but it is difficult. I still feel I ought to be doing it but I can't (*B. Hargreaves*)

I'm not well either and that's very frustrating, although I can help her (*L. Hargreaves*)

She is often agitated and it is not sparked by anything in particular. She paces around and gets very anxious. Some days you can't do anything with her. Sometimes I know what is wrong, like when she comes back from MIND and she is very agitated because she's been sat on the bus for ages. She doesn't communicate much at all. She doesn't acknowledge people, even family, although she is still quite clingy to me and gets very agitated when she thinks I will leave her. Her face was like a frightened child, that look haunted me (*G. Platt*)

I could tell when he was getting worked up and needed to go to the toilet or something. We were often in situations where we were both crying, not knowing what to do and I just had to get help, 'cause he was too upset and didn't understand what to do. I got so worn out by the incontinence, even although people were trying to help. I did a lot of learning that I had to not let him see my frustration and tears and just encouraging him all the time. A lot of the things had become too much, we both used our strong faith in Jesus and the church to help us through it. I didn't want to let him go and even now I feel like I have let him down, because I had to decide that he went. I had to realise that if he didn't go then I would have been the next to be unwell. I can mostly tell what he is trying to say even when he became unable to talk properly (*B. Taylor*)

He gets very frustrated with our youngest grandson and it is very upsetting. The little one doesn't understand. I have to separate them. With day-to-day frustrations I just can't do what I really want to any more. I feel like his mother, and that he is turning into his mother who always criticised me (*Mrs Carr*)

I read the Alzheimer's Society letter and it reassures me to know that these things are normal for the illness. I don't know how to deal with it other than to keep telling her to go into the toilet and sit down, but it goes on for ages. I just walk out a lot. I give her camomile teas and try to calm her at night (*B. Butcher*)

Theme 3: The past, the present, managing life and still having hope for the future.

This theme is about considering the actual situation, the context by which the respondents have gotten there and what they feel is in store for their future. It is important for people with dementia and their carers to be able to recognise their needs, wants and hopes for the future. This section was devised as a means of alerting people to this need and its usefulness in developing coping skills.

Q: Are you coping?

Just now we are OK. We don't need help, but don't know what will happen (*M. Hubbert*)

I think I'm getting better, sometimes I feel a bit yuck. I was down when my brother died (*D. Levers*)

It can be very difficult, when I've got to look after the tablets and all mine too (*P. Levers; Mr Levers has many health problems himself*)

At the moment we are coping (*P. and D. Levers*)

I think we are just now. Emotionally and practically 'cause carers are here (*W. Booth*)

We are coping. We know who to contact if we need help.

I am feeling OK, but am on anti-depressants now. I get highs and lows but I think I am doing OK just now. The worst thing is when I don't see anyone (*G. Platt*)

I am sort of coping (*Mrs Carr*)

I am starting to lose it a bit now. I am finding it really hard, because I feel it's my Mum and I can't turn her away, I don't want to. But I'm not a saint and if I'm not enjoying being with her, I don't want it to be like that. Sometimes she realises what she's done and she says sorry. I know she is ill but it is still very hard (*B. Butcher*)

Q: Do others help?

My family come when they can (*M. Hubbert*)

I feel sorry for him (*D. Levers*)

Neighbour is very good. Were going to put an alarm call in, but it couldn't work. We couldn't cope without them. My brother came and got me to take my tablets (*P. and D. Levers*)

Social services told me help is there, just ask. Goes to day centre one day a week. Would like that to be two days (*Anon 1*)

He stopped at day centres until he had his stroke; then they can't cope with his behaviour. His brother goes as he has it also at 41 years old (*W. Booth*)

I think the professionals should listen more to carers about whether the person is better at home or hospital. I really had to fight to have him at home and he just gave up. Only the CPN and A Society agreed he would be better at home. But by the time he came home I was exhausted by the fight. They agreed later it was right. There are not many places for people as young as him to go to (*W. Booth*)

Alzheimer's Society helps with advice about forms and benefits and meetings. Someone else who understands. CPN is there if we need him and he is very nice. We go to memory clinic for checks (*L. Hargreaves*)

Had rails and a shower put in. That helps us both. She goes to day centre one day and that gives me a break. Our daughters come round and help us a lot (*L. Hargreaves*)

It helps when friends and family visit, and I couldn't cope without the day centre three days a week, and I have a sitting service (*G. Platt*)

Now, in the home he is settled. He mostly knows me and he gives me a kiss. They are very good with him and let him do things unless he is in danger. But he has been losing a lot of weight because he just won't eat as much as he used to. His character has changed significantly, and would be awkward. Alarms and gadgets only helped so much (B. *Taylor*)

If the support I get wasn't there I wouldn't be able to cope. I think more support would help. With things like the problems with my grandson. Things like an alarm on the front door might help with him leaving the front door open all the time (*Mrs Carr*)

We have used respite twice before and it went well. So we may have to consider that on a more regular basis (B. *Butcher*)

Without the Alzheimer's Society support group, CPN and husband I couldn't continue. I wouldn't know what to do. Things that would help me are not technology because our house is quite safe and the area is too. A sitting service might be nice to let us go out for a meal on our own or something. What I have is good, but I just would like to know about the little things that happen daily, so other people in the same situation really help (B. *Butcher*)

Q: Structures/patterns and behaviours?

We get up early and usually have breakfast and the day depends on day centre or visits (M. *Hubbert*)

I get up and sorted and then get Charlie up. It takes us about 2 hours to get up. I've got a cleaner and a gardener. Go out around lunch time, have lunch, and out in afternoon for walk. Give him some jobs which he enjoys, like weeding or scrubbing bench. He gets upset to not be able to help. We are in bed by 10:30 p.m. We sleep in different rooms now and sometimes he wanders round at night but goes back when asked. Can't leave house as locks on he can't work. He doesn't try, mostly he's looking for me (*Anon 1*)

He goes for few walks a day and this keeps him calm usually. His pattern changes after respite and some days we don't know what he'll be like. Some nights he sleeps all night and others he is up all night.

I managed to get them to have carers in the respite with him and this has helped a lot with maintaining his routine and keeping him calm when he was in ward (W. *Booth*)

If she sleeps its OK, but usually I am awake a lot listening out for her (G. *Platt*)

I had to play each day by ear. I didn't know what he would want to do or agree to do each day. So I just adapted it. If he didn't accept the routine I changed it, by going out for a walk or something. Keeping to structures like day centres put a lot of stress on me to get him ready. I had to change how I talked to him, like saying someone's coming to see you rather than someone is here to fetch you. The help that you get is very good, but the problems just became too much (B. *Taylor*)

He always complies with the patterns or structures I plan, as long as we are going out. So far it's all going to plan and he does what he is asked to. He does get a bit frustrated by times and stuff (*Mrs Carr*)

We have to change the pattern daily 'cause she is different every day. Her sleeping is really bad now and she is up most of the night. Then she sleeps all day despite trying to keep her awake (B. *Butcher*)

Q: How do you get on with each other when things are tense?

We are closer now and only got married a year ago. He was deemed able to make a decision and we did it (W. *Booth*)

We loved one another and very often he would say I love you. Sometimes, it was difficult, but I had to realise that it was the disease behaving badly not him. I still loved him and I wanted to look after him, in sickness and health. He always knew me and his eyes would light up when I came in. Only when I left him with a sitter, he wouldn't talk to me when I got back. Sometimes he got aggressive when he was frustrated, but I just distracted him. Often when we went to church, even now, he was very settled (B. *Taylor*)

We have no relationship now. We don't communicate any more because he can't understand what I'm saying to him and he doesn't tell me things. It is very frustrating (*Mrs Carr*)

I don't want us to be like this. We are not able to talk and we are frustrated and nasty with each other at times. She is as glad to go to the day centre as I am too, having the break (B. *Butcher*)

Q: What is the best thing about your life just now?

Don't know really (M. *Hubbert*)

We are able to cope, but we are getting old (P. *Levers*)

We do have a good laugh. When he does something we look and both have a laugh. He hasn't lost his sense of humour. We still have a kiss and a cuddle at times (*Anon 1*)

All right (*Anon 2*)

We still love each other, he said to me this morning 'Love, love' (*W. Booth*)

There's nothing good about it (*L. Hargreaves*)

That he is settled in the nursing home. I know he is because he is not agitated when I go to see him. I think the quality of our relationship is as improved as it could be because we can just enjoy being together without the same pressures (*B. Taylor*)

That he goes to the day centre and he is always pleased to see me when I collect him (*Mrs Carr*)

I can't think of anything positive. She doesn't speak so she can't say anything nice. Occasionally she has a smile and laughs. My husband can make her laugh and she is often cheered up by ice cream, because she loves it. If she does talk it's about her mother. Sometimes after the day centre she is happy and we have a little sing-song or something. We still do things together as a family (*B. Butcher*)

Q: What is the most frustrating thing in your life just now?

To think what are we going to do, but I don't tell Pete these things, I keep it to myself (*D. Levers*)

Shaving is very frustrating, because he doesn't understand. Sometimes, I feel frustrated that we can't do what we planned for our retirement. I try not to think about it and just take each day at a time (*Anon 1*)

That I haven't got enough energy to take him out and stuff. 'Cause of my own disability I'm restricted. I feel upset and frustrated by that and do more of that with him. I just enjoy him when he comes back. We are closer now than before (*W. Booth*)

I'm not well enough to do things, nothing else (*L. Hargreaves*)

I feel irritated when I can't remember, have to ask them (*B. Hargreaves*)

She doesn't believe what we tell her (*Linda, daughter*)

I think the misunderstandings about when I would go out and he would look at me angrily. I would make a joke of it, but I had to learn to hide my feelings and he was just muddled. If I got upset it upset him (*B. Taylor*)

That I'm not living my life the way we wanted to. We wanted to tour round Europe but we can't do anything any more. It's very disappointing. The most frustrating thing for him is hard to say as he lives in his own little world (*Mrs Carr*)

The lack of sleep, incontinence and poor relationship are the hardest things for me. It feels like living with a large child and the roles are reversed. Mum gets frustrated by her own inability to do things or not knowing what is going on (*B. Butcher*)

You have to find your own way through it, but it's very hard (*B. Butcher*)

Q: *What do you think will happen next or would you like to happen next?*

Don't know what is coming (*M. Hubbert*)

I know that I can never get it out of me, never be the same again, but I have got these tablets. I don't what they are or anything. As long as we are together, and we've got a good neighbour. She's not going in a nursing home or anything like that while I can look after her. Don't what will happen if something happens to me. Always got these worries at the back of your mind (*D. Levers*)

I hope he will carry on as he is for a while. I know that next he will become more confused and less mobile and need a lot more care at home. I will keep him here as long as I can (*W. Booth*)

We will get more help if we need it. I think we need a home help (*L. Hargreaves*)

I wouldn't mind if we had a cleaner (*B. Hargreaves*)

My mum thinks it's a baby sitter and won't have it (*Linda, daughter*)

I am going to have to make a decision about long-term care. I want her at home just now. I want my kids to get our money anyway, not to pay for care. I think it will be when she can't walk I may have to (*G. Platt*)

When I look at the others there doesn't seem to be any set patterns so I don't know. I hope he won't have to go into a home, but if he got incontinent I think he would have to go. I would feel a failure if he had to. I feel that I should look after him, for better or for worse. I hope I can cope till the end (*Mrs Carr*)

If it continues the way it's going then I think she will end up in a home. Maybe respite would delay it a bit, but I think it will come (*B. Butcher*)

PART 2

Practical aspects of care: incorporating theory with the lived experience

CHAPTER 5

Psychological and emotional effects of dementia and memory loss

Learning points on the effects of psychological issues:

■ Fear and its effect on developing coping strategies
■ Depression and its influence on dementia
■ How we can help ourselves and each other by practical guidance and emotional support techniques

Harris and Durkin (2002; cited in Norman and Ryrie, 2004, pp. 572–3) identified key adapting strategies used by the sample group in their study. These people successfully managed to cope and adapt their approach to the many problems they faced. In reference to psychological effects they identified the following as a means of dealing with these effects:

■ *Acceptance and ownership* as a method of alleviating any feelings of guilt for not achieving or doing something wrong.
■ *Disclosure* to other people outside the family allowed the carers to express their feelings openly and without having to restrain frustration and embarrassment.
■ *Positive attitude and self-acceptance* meant that people were able to face the effects of dementia and how it affected them individually with a more positive thought process.
■ *Role relinquishment and replacement* offered an alternative to just accepting the loss of a person, to finding a new personality and its positives.
■ *Innovative techniques* and use of technology helped with many practical issues and could perhaps with further study be examined as to whether it influenced confidence and self-esteem.
■ *Fluidity* meant that acceptance of the daily progression of the disease allowed people to see it as part of their life and offered them a semblance of normality.
■ *Utilising proactive skills* like changing routines to suit the issues of that day rather than just carrying on with a detrimental pattern. This would again alleviate the stress of daily conflict or distress.

- *Connecting with past activities* helped people to identify things they did in the past which should be adapted to now, and therefore present them with some meaningful activity.
- *Anticipatory adaptation* means the preparation for the future, and many people in this study found it useful to begin adapting for what could potentially happen before it did.
- *Altruistic acts* seemed to offer people the chance to feel as though they were still a contributor to society and could still be part of the community.
- *Holistic practices* like yoga were found to be enjoyable and could be another area for further research into any benefits.
- *Spirituality* provided many of the study respondents with a means of support, and they found this very beneficial.

Many of these key themes have also been found in the interviews for this book, which can only enhance the credibility of the small samples used in both. However, there are of course many people in the UK and the rest of the world who have different experiences of living with dementia and would add even more to this guidance if they were approached.

This chapter will concentrate on themes identified as affecting a person's emotional and psychological well-being.

This section will now try to offer some guidance on how people can deal with these issues based on current knowledge of the respondents themselves and that of the theory offered at present.

Fear of dementia

Fear was identified by many respondents, and if we consider dementia and its effect on a person who has little support we can begin to appreciate just how debilitating a diagnosis of this nature must be.

> I cried a lot. I thought they were going to come and take me away. I didn't think anything was wrong.

This person was anguished by the thought of the unknown and possibly some missing information about what it means to have dementia. It is appropriate to assume that non-professional people will not be aware of the reality of dementia or of the services and support which will be made available to them at the initial stages of diagnosis. It is therefore easy to assume that professionals should expect that informing a person of the diagnosis will vary with patient/client and will require individualised approaches. One carer commented that the neurologist who gave them the diagnosis was 'very abrasive' and ignored the obvious distress expressed by the couple. Another carer explained that her mother was very defensive about questions that she could not answer and the interview became, in her view, of little use. One sufferer expressed his concern in the extreme. He assumed that this diagnosis meant that he would die and the carer felt that in the future avoidance of the subject was the best way to alleviate this distress.

Overall, the anticipation of what is to come when given a diagnosis like dementia is bound to cause both realistic and/or irrational fears and worries. The role of the professional carer in this instance is to accept this need and provide emotional support to the person diagnosed and the informal carer involved. This approach of assuming the need for support will mean that people are not assumed to be coping, thus opening the doors to the value of professional assessment and support.

Non-professional carers have a different role in this aspect of care. They not only have to deal with their own fears and anxieties about what will happen next, but:

> I felt like my life was over, I had no life of my own any more.

The need for carers to access support is paramount to a successful relationship with the sufferer, and this will be explored in the chapter on support.

Meanwhile, the carer has the responsibility of day-to-day care and needs to learn to adapt to living in this way.

Many of the carers talked about the time of diagnosis as one of enormous stress and worry:

> Couldn't take it in at first

> I couldn't really believe it at first, felt like it was happening to someone else.

> When they told what was wrong I was quite shocked, and I kept it to myself. I didn't want to admit what was wrong. Took me a while to accept it, still thought it was his age until things got a bit worse

> Numb, surprised, emotional, not wanting to face the truth.... We went home and tried to think what will we do, then we tried to forget about it but couldn't

> We tried to forget but couldn't 'cause of the misunderstandings

In these statements it is apparent that denial plays a big part in the period of time around the initial diagnosis. The concerns that people have are usually based on a need to know what is wrong, yet a need to pretend that it is not happening because it feels so devastating. Perhaps the non-professional's disadvantage of having a limited knowledge about dementia leads them to this fear and devastation. However, it is also a realistic perspective about a condition which affects a person in every possible part of their life in a very distressing way. As expected, feelings of devastation were also expressed:

> I was devastated. How were we going to cope? I was on my own.

This carer was feeling particularly vulnerable due to her own disability restrictions and felt completely unprepared for the onset of dementia in her husband.

Not understanding the diagnosis can also unearth deep-rooted beliefs about its origin and possible path and many people may find it too difficult to accept the actual diagnosis until the symptoms progress beyond any other explanation:

> I thought I was going daft, I didn't like that but got used to it and you learn to live with it.

This sufferer explained her acceptance of her path to certain extent once she had entered into it and realised that she was still able to do things, albeit in a different way.

> My husband had no recognition of it at all. He asked once what Alzheimer's is, but didn't understand.

The assumption that a person does not understand can be misleading. It may be in this case that the sufferer had connected with the diagnosis but was unable to communicate his fear or need to know more effectively. When he was given information he was unable to understand it, or accept it. The issue here is that he asked about it, indicating that he had thought about Alzheimer's, and this may have been causing him anxiety.

The feelings of insecurity and fear were vividly apparent at this stage of each of the respondents' journeys into life with dementia, and this led many to begin to question their future:

> All these years she's been looking after me, now we have to look after each other.

> When it was all happening I was lost, bewildered and angry. Maureen did everything and I didn't know how to do anything – cook, shop or anything. Everything was blown apart.

> The problem is that you don't get enough information, because they don't know I suppose what will happen, but it would really help.

When I look at others there doesn't seem to be any set patterns, so I don't know what will happen in the future.

I should like to look after him till the end, I hope I can cope.

If it continues the way it's going then I think she will end up in a home.

Sufferers and carers alike described very depressed feelings associated with anxiety about the symptoms, but also with guilt about future decisions to be made. Many people with dementia are indeed diagnosed with depression; some are treated and some not. Carers also suffer from these distressing symptoms and need support. However, the availability of this support seems to be variable and inconsistent. Within this small group it is quite apparent that both carers and sufferers could benefit greatly from some kind of treatment or therapy for depression or at the very least a low mood.

I was very depressed and cried a lot (*sufferer*)

He was not depressed about it.

He said it was getting too much for him.

She was very depressed.

Without the onset of dementia 9.2% of the population under 64 years old will suffer from mixed anxiety and depression (Office for National Statistics, 2000), and of those over 64 years old 6–7% will suffer from the same (Office for National Statistics, 2003). These figures offer us an insight into just how common depression is among the general population, and it is important to remember that people with one problem can have another: dementia does not preclude someone from becoming depressed and needing help with the problems of depression as well as the dementia.

Depression is described as a chronic illness (DSM-IV, 1994):

depressed mood along with a set of additional symptoms persisting over time and leading to disruptions and impairment in functioning

The problem with this medical description is that it offers a similar path of symptoms to those found in dementia, and often, as a result of this, depression continues undiagnosed, and therefore untreated.

I thought it was depression at first, 'cause her Mum had just died.

How we can help ourselves and each other

- **Information giving and finding**: As expressed in the comments, people felt bewildered and unprepared for what was inevitable in their lives and they believed this was partly due to a lack of knowledge about it. This can be remedied by professionals giving out information through health promotion exercises and strategies, such as local organisations and leaflet distribution. Carers can find this information before professional intervention if they go to local health facilities (e.g. GP surgeries) or search on the Internet. Once professional care is in progress, the sufferer and carer may need more in-depth information about the particular diagnosis, which can be found in specialist organisations like the Alzheimer's Society, the Huntington's Disease Association, the CJD Alliance, MIND and the Mental Health Foundation. Also, in the general literature there are books of people's experiences of living with dementia, such as Miller (2003) and Bryden (2005). It is also important for people to be able to read and be told about different approaches to dementia. The medical explanation and treatment are only one facet of this problem and sufferers and carers need to know that there are social, psychological and practical implications which they need support with also. Many of the organisations identified here do offer this kind of guidance and their contact details are all offered in Chapter 6. Alternative explanations are offered in Chapter 2.
- **Individualised approach**: The need to see dementia as devastating and yet liveable is perhaps the most important aspect of learning to adapt to it in people's lives. To assume that it affects everyone in the same way and only be able to see it from a negative perspective often leads professionals, carers and sufferers alike to lose the drive to see the person still living. Despite the popular conception of dementia, it does not mean that the person has joined the living dead. It does mean, however, that they have changed significantly and need to adapt to a new way of life that they would most certainly not have chosen, but are nevertheless faced with. In order that this change of lifestyle can take place it is essential that they and people around them still value them and their contribution to making plans, either on a simple daily task basis or on making life decisions. Therefore the ability to see the person as changing and in need of enormous support to do so may help carers to accept the changes as a distressing but necessary part of all their lives. The alternative is to let go of any connection and assume that they have left their lives before they actually have.
- **Dealing with denial**: Denial plays a big part in the initial stages of any life problems or worries, and being given a diagnosis of dementia is no exception. The people involved in being given this diagnosis may find that their fears are compounded by the lack of awareness (or alternatively full aware-

ness) of what this means and therefore reject the idea in an effort to avoid the distress that goes with such situations. Perhaps we should consider this a normal response (indeed it is), but it soon becomes a hindrance to learning to live with the problems. If denial is continual then people cannot accept the problem and then find support to live with their new situation. So that individuals can overcome this it is important to ensure that diagnosis is discussed in depth and with the individualised approach discussed above. This will mean that people can connect with problems directly related to them. Not understanding the diagnosis is an obvious problem for the sufferer, and sometimes for the carer, but it should be dealt with as yet another problem which needs to be tackled and not just left alone. The development of individualised communication with the person can help them to understand to different extents what is happening to them. As a result, many anxieties and fears can be either allayed or empathised with and supported.

- **Changing lifestyles**: This is probably by far the most significant issue in the early days of dementia. Many of the interviewees gave us an insight into just how scary this prospect actually is. People felt unable to change and some are not even aware of the need to. The result of not being aware or of how to change is often at the root of frustration and friction between sufferers and carers and its effect can be seen in the negative alteration of feelings about each other. Sufferers have to be able to adapt to their changing world if they are to be able to live in it with some quality of life. So that they can do that it is important to change routines and daily patterns to suit the needs of that day. This may be a very difficult task for people who have a certain way of life which they enjoy, like going on regular holidays or socialising regularly. The continuation of previous patterns will often lead to conflict and feelings of resentment towards those around them. Ultimately this is in itself very upsetting, but it may only take a small change to overcome this. For example, instead of going on holiday alone, find companions who understand the problems, or have friends visit at home rather than going out to unfamiliar places to prevent disorientation and agitation. Couples may benefit from time away from each other by asking a friend to help, or by using professional carers in the form of day centres or sitting services, which are provided by all social services departments.
- **Learn new skills**: In many cases of couples affected by dementia the carer becomes depended upon for all the household jobs and all the sufferer's personal care as well. To be able to deal with this it may be necessary to learn how to cook, clean or shop. Some people have never handled the finances of the family and may need to learn very quickly how to access their money and pay bills, sometimes first having to find out what bills there actually are. For individuals to do this it is important to remember that it won't all happen at once and that a gradual adaptation to these life skills will be possible. Perhaps the use of books and reading will help, but equally family and friends

may be able to offer guidance. Learning to cook could even be seen as a positive outcome, which if time is available to attend a local college course can offer some much needed socialising time and enjoyment. However, it is necessary to remain realistic, and many new carers cannot spare the time to attend such activities. Therefore the use of learning manuals and other people's support is indeed a very positive way to develop these skills.

- **Learn to communicate feelings**: The carer and sufferer need to be able to communicate with each other effectively. The spoken word is by far the preferred human means of contact and is therefore unfortunately assumed to be the only way. For people with dementia, whose ability to talk about things is usually affected early on in the progress of the problems, this can mean that any spoken communication they offer is treated as not relevant or lacking understanding. There are in fact many ways for people to communicate, and this is evident in the population of people with hearing or speech difficulties by use of other languages, e.g. Makaton. Also, if we consider babies and the development of sign language for them before they learn to talk, we can see examples of how just some people have overcome this problem. There are also other means of communication available to the person with dementia, in the form of facial expression, body posture and mood. For example, if a person begins to cry, it can be assumed that they are upset by something, whether they have dementia or not. If they are laughing or grinning, or even just smiling, then that is also a telling expression of feeling: they like what is happening. The history of a person's life can also help to decipher what they are trying to say or want. Simply by being aware that they have a background in cleaning for a living may explain repetitive dusting and moving of items. The ability to communicate with the individual helps the carer to accept that this person has still got stuff to do and say – they just need to be listened to. Developing a realistic awareness of the sufferer's understanding is the difference between maintaining contact and becoming strangers.

- **Look out for depression**: If the carer or sufferer has suffered from depression in the past then they are automatically at higher risk of developing it again under this pressure. Generally, however, everyone in such a stressful situation is vulnerable to becoming depressed and should be monitored for the following signs:

  - *Emotions*: Sadness, tearfulness, loss of pleasure in usual activities, feeling hopeless and guilty
  - *Motivation*: Increased dependency on others, low energy and fatigue and poor concentration
  - *Cognitive*: Negative expectations and self-image, difficulty making decisions which would have been easy before, preoccupation with illness and any interest expressed in self-harm or suicide

- *Psychomotor*: Changes in appetite or sleep and consequent weight loss or sleep deprivation, reduced sexual drive and function, early wakening and sleeping day instead of night
- *Physical*: Changes in body patterns like constipation/diarrhoea, stomach cramps, nausea or irregular menstrual cycles

If any of these symptoms become persistent and occur together then it is very important to seek help from the medical profession, counsellors or support organisations. Left untreated, depression can cause a person to feel so distressed that they may even feel they want to die. Apart from the severity of what it could lead to, it is not necessary for people to suffer in this way. The support and help that they get can alleviate the desperate feelings and the sometimes difficult to handle behaviour associated with it. During the time waiting to be seen by a professional it is important for the person suffering the depression and the carer to be able to talk about their feelings. Just the acceptance of the distress can open up a channel of communication which may lead to talking about how support can be offered. Sometimes if people don't know what to say just allowing each other to cry or offer comfort can help. Otherwise start with 'How are you feeling?' They may even tell you.

Develop self-esteem and feelings of well-being by encouraging achievable tasks or activities. Stimulate the imagination by offering different means of expression (such as drawing) and challenge preconceptions by remembering that the sufferer does still have abilities, although they may be much limited from before (Craig and Killick, 2004).

Personality changes

Learning points on the effect of changing personalities:

- Changing personalities and the associated emotional turmoil
- How we can help ourselves and each other by identifying these issues and learning to deal with them effectively

The change of personality in dementia is an inevitable consequence and its effect is often the most difficult to bear for those people involved who value each other's personal attributes and values. It is important to remember that these changes in perspective happen in everyone's lives simply with the passage of time, but for those experiencing the severe and sometimes shocking changes found in sufferers of dementia this is a very pronounced and damaging problem.

Often people who were previously very compliant and generous in conversation become evasive and argumentative:

> Mum got really defensive when asked assessment questions 'cause she didn't know the answers.

The need of the individual in this situation is understanding and acceptance that they are scared of the fact that they cannot answer a relatively simple question. The assumption that they are just being difficult and argumentative can only serve to fuel the frustration and resentment already possibly present in the relationship.

The person will change and in many cases the disorientation of the symptoms will lead the person to become, hostile, aggressive, suspicious, angry and defensive:

> He got so frustrated at times and angry. He didn't know what was going on and become frustrated with everyone.

> He was so upset by it that I had to just let him do it.

> She started accusing people of doing things to her and when reminiscing with a friend this became worse.

> She started thinking she was in her dad's house and trying to throw me out.

> She was a very active person before, holidaying on her own after Dad died, so she wanted to continue and I had to stop her.

> We used to go out all the time, but he wouldn't cope with these things any more.

> She thinks we are all against her and doing things behind her back. We do tell her everything but she forgets.

> She doesn't remember us, won't even answer to Mum.

> He lost his license and now complains constantly that he never drives.

> I get frustrated and very upset when I can't see what to do next, and I have to ask them.

> We don't communicate any more because he can't understand what I'm saying to him and he doesn't tell me things. It is very frustrating.

> His character changed significantly and would be awkward.

The effect of personality change is evident here and seems to suggest that the most detrimental aspect of it results from the reduced ability of sufferers to be able to communicate their feelings, needs and general wants in life. Carers are often left feeling resentful of the loss of a person they knew well and depended on for a certain regularity in their lives.

The changes mean that either has to be able to understand the other's perspective.

How we can help each other or ourselves

- **Accept the change**: Ultimately, trying to resist the inevitable changes of life with dementia from a previous lifestyle will only serve to increase dissatisfaction and frustration. If the sufferer and carer can begin to understand that there is nothing they can do to stop change then they can begin to adapt to whatever that change may be. The constant use of communicating with each other is a very useful way to keep up to date with the sometimes daily and other times slow progression and consequent differences in life. Just spending time talking or communicating by other means, like interpreting behaviour and facial expressions discussed earlier, or drawing pictures or writing poems etc., are all very useful ways of understanding the constantly changing position of each person involved. The resolve offered by accepting the situation and then learning to adapt to it seems altogether less exhausting than fighting a losing battle on a daily basis. This acceptance should not be seen as a 'giving up the fight' response, but rather an acknowledgement of what the fight actually is. The struggle is not with whether we can control these alterations in our lives, because that is inevitable, but more about how resourceful we are in adapting to them.
- **Grieve the loss of the lifestyle not the person**: It is important to remember that the sufferer is still there and that to discount them as not part of the conscious world, or childlike, or the living dead is not only disrespectful but also potentially disheartening if they can sense this kind of negativity towards them in any way. In acceptance of these problems and changes there will be feelings of loss. People can and should be able to grieve the loss of anything including losing the opportunity to carry out previous life plans, like travelling or socialising or taking up a hobby or just simply spending time enjoying relaxing or exciting activities. Whatever the loss, it will be difficult to accept, but possible if adaptation is an option open to them. The personality lost is of course very distressing and feels like the person themselves has gone. If we consider the whole person then perhaps there is a way to understand that it is parts of them which have changed or disappeared, sometimes replaced by undesirable traits, but it is still possible to recognise some of the remaining familiar aspects. For example, a person with dementia may not recognise anyone formally by name or even acknowledge them,

but if responses are watched carefully, more often than not the sufferer will be seen to be familiar with certain people and more content in that company.

■ **Be realistic about the relationship**: The relationship that is affected by someone having dementia should not be assumed to be one of great closeness before the onset of these particular problems. Dementia affects people in difficult relationships as well as strong close ones. If we assume that all families are the same then we are not offering individual support, and any help offered may inflame old problems and conflicts. It is important to be aware of the basis of any interactions and relationships so that whatever its premise the sufferer and/or carer are supported. For example, a husband and wife may have been going through difficulties in their marriage which led to conflict prior to the onset of dementia. To offer this couple supported holidays together would be of little use, whereas counselling and relationship support might help. Alternatively, just time apart may appease conflicts. Parent and children relationships may be full of friction and need enormous support in this way before even starting on the symptoms of the dementia.

■ **Communicate on a different level**: If acceptance, grieving and realistic approaches are used then the next task is to try to learn how to communicate with this person in an effective way. As discussed previously, there are many ways to communicate with people other than talking. Use alternatives:

- *Use cue cards*: 'The toilet', pictures of the activity or item, short concise reminders like 'close the door', name badges and orientation boards.
- *Watch and familiarise self with facial expressions, body postures, general movements and demeanours*. Recording these regularly can help to build up a pattern of what they might mean by relating them to what is going on whenever they carry out this expression or behaviour.
- *Shouting and aggression cannot be dealt with by reciprocating*. Be aware of the frustration behind it and try to console the person rather than enter into an irrational argument or power struggle.
- *The professional carer should seek to understand the person's history* in an effort to understand their interpretation of events in the present. This will help the pair to find common ground and be able to grasp each other's perspective.
- *Develop awareness of own expressions and behaviours*: People are often unaware of the effect, or even the presence, of a scowl or facial look of discouragement. This can be very powerful to the person with limited ability to understand instruction. Remember that communication goes two ways and the sufferer has to be able to read the carer's expressions also. The relevant expression at the time is important and to be able to

understand each other carers have to learn about their own communications and the effect they have on others as well as being able to read the others. This can be done by asking other people to help to identify mannerisms. Make a point of recording what you were doing when the person reacted in the way they did. This can help to identify appropriate or not so appropriate responses.

- **Change interpretation of behaviour**: Learning to understand the behaviour or responses offered by each person involved is the basic premise of 'person-centred care' (Kitwood, 1997). In understanding the behaviour and then responding to the reason for it, it may be that it can be prevented or appeased by just accepting and not challenging the person. It is part of Kitwood's philosophy that the reasons behind behaviour always explain them, and therefore we can adjust our environment and approaches in an effort to prevent difficult-to-manage behaviours from occurring in the first place. This theory has been very popular in the professional circles involved in care of a person with dementia and even if it does not achieve this goal it does offer people a chance to be treated with respect and dignity. It is essential to meet the previous challenges on this list of how to help, to be able to offer person-centred care. It is equally important to remember that in individual perspectives people may have behavioural traits which have never conformed to societal rules, and therefore will not now. The person with dementia may have been a very disruptive person before its onset. Understanding why they were this way may be impossible to investigate or appreciate. The concern here is how this person is understood now. In the context of the past it is possible to explain behaviour but not always to understand it. Once again we come back to the basic issue of not assuming anything and being able to adapt to the routine, environment and communication of that individual person.
- **Get emotional support**: At difficult times in life most people have someone they can talk to about problems. If this is possible now, then use this resource to express feelings and frustrations outside the circle of people immediately affected. Many people do not have this luxury in the first place and often the person with dementia is the one they may have confided in before. This leaves people with a great big missing link in their support network. The sufferers themselves lose the emotional support of relatives or friends. As they become more distant as the problems persist, there is generally a lack of ability to express the anger, frustration and fear in a safe place. Use the Health Service and social services support professionals, such as nurses, social workers and carers, to get this help. Other organisations like the Alzheimer's Society and MIND also offer counselling services and support groups.

Changes in the relationship

Learning points on the effect of the changes in relationships:

- Changes in relationships between anyone involved with a person with dementia and the ultimate feelings of loss
- Sexuality, sex and emotional attachment as an issue
- Life plans and the challenge of dealing with changing expectations
- How we can help ourselves and each other by acceptance and learning a new way of life and different responses

The changes in a relationship are significant for all people involved with a person who has dementia. It is one of the most distressing effects of this problem as it can lead to feelings of hostility, suspicion and isolation. The person with dementia is responding to many changes in their mental state. The person involved – spouse, child, friend, partner, colleague, neighbour or any other – is left wondering why they are behaving in this way and how they can help. The interviews demonstrate that this change in the relationship can be very negative, but a relationship of a different form can be developed.

The following quotes show people's feelings, which suggest frustration and general sadness. These are normal and understandable in such a time of stress and anxiety. Most of the carers were able to explain these feelings clearly and have all had time enough to think about them. For people just entering this way of life it can be a time of feeling guilty for having them in the first place. Remember, feelings are always important and valid – the only issue is how you deal with them.

> 'Cause we couldn't talk I got frustrated. We used to fight all the time. He just shut himself away.

> We had always been really close and then I felt she started caring for me less and less. I thought we were just growing apart.

> I just started to feel that he wasn't my husband any more, not the man I married, and not a man I liked very much any more.

> Because I had to do everything I got tired and then we ended up arguing a lot.

> We fell out a lot because I didn't know then.

> She never talks about my Dad, only her mum and sisters. That upsets me.

> It upsets me when he snaps at me.

I got so worn out by the incontinence, even although people were trying to help me.

We have no relationship now. We don't communicate any more because he can't understand what I'm saying to him, and he doesn't tell me things.

For young or adult children the change in relationship is immense. It is difficult to imagine how the person who taught you how to behave is now in need of your total understanding and care.

It's my Mum and I can't turn her away, I don't want to. But I'm not a saint and if I'm not enjoying being with her, I don't want it to be like that.

The suspicious nature of some people with dementia can also be very disappointing and lead to further feelings of resentment.

She doesn't believe what we tell her.

Many families find that the sufferer becomes very intolerant of young children, and grandchildren are often the victim of hostility. The family can often become embroiled in lots of consoling of children who don't understand and become upset by the response they receive from a previously friendly grandparent.

He gets very frustrated with our youngest grandson. The little one doesn't understand and it is very upsetting.

We went out one day with the grandchildren and he was very sharp with them.

However, despite all these negative changes in the relationships there are ways to adapt and change it so that we still get something from it. Most people's resentment of the relationship is because of the loss of one which used to feel good and happy.

I don't want us to be like this, we are not able to talk, and get very frustrated and nasty with each other.

It is important to remember that the need to grieve for what the relationship was is essential to be able to accept the good in what it has become, as can be seen in the following carers' quotes.

He was crying a lot, we ended up crying together.

He enjoys the day centre, and often says he wishes I could come.

Mostly he's looking for me.

We loved one another and very often we would say I love you. I still loved him and wanted to look after him, in sickness and in health.

We are closer now and only got married a year ago.

We still love each other, he said to me this morning: love, love.

We do have a laugh together, he hasn't lost his sense of humour.

I think the quality of our relationship has improved, since in the nursing home, as we can just enjoy each other without all the pressures.

He goes to the day centre and is always pleased to see me when I collect him.

Sometimes after the day centre she is happy and we have a little sing-song. We still do things as a family.

I just enjoy him when he comes back. We are closer now than before.

We should also consider how the sufferer may be feeling about this relationship change. It is easy to assume that they don't feel the loss or lose any compassion for the other person, but this feeling is perhaps present, just not being communicated.

I do think what are we going to do, but don't tell him that (*sufferer*)

I feel sorry for him (*sufferer*)

Sexuality

The sexual relationship of any couple is different, and sexuality is not just about the act of sex. It involves the affection and general companionship of each other. When someone has dementia one of the skills they may lose is the ability to initiate an activity, including being passionate or affectionate. This does not mean that they don't feel it, just simply that they cannot express it in the way that they may have done previously.

She was started on anti-depressants and they helped her a lot. It really lifted her spirits and the physical side of our relationship returned.

He mostly knows me and he gives me a kiss.

We still have a kiss and a cuddle now and again.

Nay (2003) also identified key areas of sexuality for older people as look-ing nice, cuddling, touching and just being with the opposite sex. Sexuality is discussed as a central aspect of being a human and encompasses sex, gender, identities and roles, sexual orientation, eroticism, pleasure, intimacy and repro-duction by the World Health Organization, although not as a definition but as guidance on professional perspectives (World Health Organization, 2006).

The sufferer's choice in how they present themselves in a physical way is usually limited in this situation because of practical reasons. This lack of con-trol over the ability to define yourself to those around you could have a negative effect on a person's self-esteem and confidence. The ability to present ourselves to the rest of the world in the way we see as appropriate is an important part of self-identity and most people with dementia depend very much on carers making choices that are similar to, if not the same, as they would have made. The many issues of a person's dignity are to be examined when looking at per-sonal care and hygiene, such as going to the toilet. It must be a difficult change of lifestyle to accept anyone taking you to the toilet and cleaning you.

I choose his clothes and help him dress.

He had bowel problems and got really irritated by me taking him there.

He does what I tell him.

Relationships vary and there is no standard for how these kinds of things are dealt with other than to understand that everyone involved will have different needs and has to resolve the issue of sexuality accordingly.

We sleep in different rooms now.

Life plans

Another loss felt by sufferers and carers is that of their plans. Many people have lots of plans for what they will do when retired or when they have time, and others expect that they will tick along and continue as they were. It is very disappointing to find that in fact all this planning and anticipation for relaxing or exciting times in our lives will not only have to change but may not happen at all.

I feel frustrated that we can't do what we planned for our retirement.

I can't take him out 'cause of my own disability.

That we're not living the life we wanted to. We wanted to tour Europe but we can't do anything any more. It's very disappointing.

As a result of the practical and emotional changes and restrictions on the sufferers' and carers' lives, people end up feeling isolated. This is a very vulnerable time and it is important to be able to see that there are alternatives to just suffering and just caring in order to survive it well.

I saw a woman from the Alzheimer's association and remember telling her I felt my life was over, I had no life of my own any more.

The worst thing is when I don't see anyone.

I keep it to myself (*sufferer*)

The creation of dependence is one which changes the relationship beyond recognition. It is this change which affects people in a way that they may have never considered. The shock of dementia conjures up the feelings of loss but does little to prepare people for the new nursing skills they will have to learn. Dependence is, however, controllable in certain ways and is found to some degree to be influenced by the progression of the sufferer's symptoms and the coping skills of the carer.

Once he knew what it was, he got so that he needed looking after.

I do everything for her, wash her and cut up food. She tells me when she needs to go to the toilet.

It is possible to maintain the sufferer's activity and input into daily tasks by changing the emphasis or routine.

Give him some jobs, like weeding or scrubbing the bench. He gets upset when not able to help.

How we can help ourselves and each other

■ **Accept feelings as normal**: Understand the implications of dementia as beyond your control. This may help you to see the problems you face with a sense of relief: it is nobody's fault! All the feelings that form the response of the carer are simply a result of what is happening and the enormity of these changes in lives. It is easy to accept the burden of guilt and assume that if the person with dementia had not eaten an unhealthy diet then they would have been fine. The fact is that research has so far not pinpointed a controllable and definitive cause for any type of dementia. The ability to use emotionally supportive people at this time may help a person to talk about these feelings of guilt or anger, which sometimes helps to put them into perspective and understand the reality of the situation. Professional support can also help with this: counsellors, nurses, social workers, support groups and doctors.

- **Learn to understand the reason for the changes**: Where does dementia come from and why does it affect people differently? The main points or issues in this text are about this very concern and the individuality of each person's experience of dementia. Despite the common patterns of the symptoms, the people themselves are different and therefore respond in variable ways to the changes. This is a good time to start trying to get to grips with the person being cared for in a more intimate way. The use of history-taking and reminiscing can often help carers to establish the person's likes and dislikes more accurately. However, it is important to remember that, as with anyone, people change during their lifetimes, and something that a person enjoyed many years ago may not be something they enjoy now. Always establish the present likes and dislikes in combination with building up a picture of their life story. Also, when considering such techniques it has been found in the past that some people find reminiscing very distressing. They may be asked to recall very difficult periods in their lives, and this is upsetting. The carer should be prepared for a range of emotions and should adapt to the person's needs today. Family or friend carers can also try this technique by trying to talk about memories and discussing periods of their lives for enjoyment.

- **Encourage children to be involved**: The family unit often contains a few children here and there. It would be impossible for contact to continue between the sufferer and the children without them noticing that something is wrong. Therefore it is perhaps a good idea to explain the reasons for these changes in the adult so that some kind of understanding can be achieved.

> Always remember that it is dementia that is making them behave in that way and that it's not your fault. All you can do is your best. (Mental Health Foundation, 2005)

There has been some literature written for children which explains the problems and tries to alleviate their worries and anxieties by explaining the effects of dementia to them (Shriver, 2004; Fine, 2002; Gilliard, 1995). There are also fact sheets and a video to be found through local Alzheimer's Societies which may help with this process.

- **Learn to explain and repeat**: The acceptance of the changes already discussed will prepare the carer for this task with a lessened level of frustration. Essentially the aim is to communicate with the person, and this requires key skills when the ability of the individual responding is impaired (National Institute of Aging, 2002):

  - Choose simple words and short sentences and use a gentle, calm tone of voice.

- Avoid using baby talk; this will only add insult to injury in their already fragile sensibilities and disorientation.
- Minimise distractions when talking (turn down the television for example); this will mean that the information can be concentrated on.
- Gain the attention of the person by saying their name, getting eye contact or holding their hand.
- Allow time for them to respond, then establish their understanding of the conversation.
- Prompt responses to help the conversation be two-way and therefore have more impact on them.

■ **Set boundaries**: To maintain a sense of individuality and self-esteem it may be necessary for carers to set some boundaries as to the particular tasks they undertake with the person with dementia. The use of professional support may help to alleviate issues around toileting and intimate personal care if these are affecting the person in a distressing way. Professional carers have to set boundaries around their own emotional involvement to prevent creating a potentially damaging dependence on them. If the boundaries are not set then people involved become confused about the help they can receive and may find it hard to ask whether a personal relationship has been established. It is possible to show compassion and understanding without becoming part of the trauma themselves. Simply establishing the role of the carers helps to alleviate these pressures and thus enhances the time that is spent together.

■ **Accept changes and re-plan**: The devastation of the changes in these lives is almost incomprehensible, but it has been shown by the people interviewed that lives can be adapted and made to fit. It would be a futile battle to continue trying to achieve some goals set previously. Perhaps the next challenge for the people involved is to change these plans to something that is realistic for them and their new situation. However, it is not easy to let go of aspirations and dreams and it is difficult to think of new ones when under such pressure all the time. The acceptance of the need to do so is the first step, followed by learning to move on the next. Again, professionals can help with this kind of planning by offering a listening ear and some encouragement to continue. The individuals could always start with simple things like just getting out the house to go to a local social event once a week. There is no need to plan a skiing trip in a place with nursing support, but it is possible to have holidays in certain circumstances. Voluntary organisations can often help to assess whether this is realistic for the individual situation and help to plan it.

■ **Break the cycle of dependence**: It has been shown that there are cycles of dependence in caring relationships and that these can lead to deterioration in the skill and ability of those being cared for. Despite this, the need for care is obvious in many different ways and should of course be attended to with compassion and assistance. Breaking this cycle is not an attempt to punish or humiliate the person with dementia, but more to empower them and potentially increase their self-esteem and confidence. This is assumed, in turn, to maintain abilities for as long as possible, which will mean less dependence and stress on the carer in the long run. How this can be done is the part where the carer has to learn to allow the person to try tasks rather than assuming that they can't do it. This requires patience and understanding, as their potentially slow thinking processes are trying to work through the activity. It is also necessary to prioritise which tasks need to take place at a certain time. The carer will benefit greatly from being able to be flexible and changing routines daily if necessary. The need to have a bath every night may not be as important as the pair having some time together and trying to communicate. This of course depends on the individual and what they feel or want at the time, as well as the practicalities of needing to get somewhere in a hurry.

- **Respect the individual right to be a sexual being**: Respect the person's right to be a man or women and to maintain their sexual orientation. Whilst accepting the right to maintain a sexual identity and activity, this must be weighed against the risk of abuse. Vulnerability is a key issue for people with dementia and memory problems and sexual identity could be a means of abuse. However, this can be minimised, as can any risk of abuse, by careful monitoring of behaviour and looking for signals or signs of distress associated with any particular person or action.

Use of touching, counselling, compassion and empathy are key characteristics of careering for another person. Positive use of these skills and attitudes can be used in a non-sexual way to ensure that people continue to control this aspect of their lives.

Carer stress

Learning points on the effects of caring on carers

- Identifying and acknowledging the implications of dealing with carer stress
- Spirituality and its use as a means of support for the person with dementia and for carers
- Making decisions about long-term care
- How we can help ourselves and each other

She cried when I said she should see a doctor; she thought it was just me getting on at her.

I get upset and frustrated when I can't see what I need to do next and I have to ask them. They are very good and they help me but it's difficult, I still feel I ought to be doing it myself (*sufferer*)

Her face was like a frightened child, that look haunted me.

The most frustrating thing for him is hard to say as he lives in his own little world.

Mum gets frustrated by her own inability to do things or by not knowing what is going on.

I think the most frustrating thing is the misunderstandings about when I wanted to go out, and he would look at me angrily.

I'm not well enough to do things (*sufferer*)

Many of these comments demonstrate the amount of distress associated with a caring role. It is also very evident in research that carer stress is a major reason for relationship breakdown or the onset of poor care conditions. Professional carers can use measurement tools to assess the level of stress in a caring relationship. This can help to identify those at risk of the negative effects of extreme stress and pressure by simply identifying it early and putting in place adequate support. The professional can be influential in this aspect of care by developing a strong relationship which is built on the experience of each other's reactions, feelings and needs. The use of this individual awareness could mean the ability to identify carer stress at its onset and therefore prevent the problems occurring. Alternatively, it could be used to identify a crisis and clarify the person's needs at the time more accurately. Zarit *et al.* (1987) identify a stress reduction model for working with carers which includes information-giving and promoting problem-solving with the family. This basis to any approach can offer an enhanced professional relationship which is easily utilised as required. The person with dementia also expresses stress here, and it is obvious that both parties are feeling the enormous pressure of becoming dependant on each other for support.

Depression is a common problem for both the person with dementia and the carer. The need to be aware of this potential problem is vital in being able to prevent or identify it early to alleviate the problems it causes.

We cried together.

Things got too much and I couldn't do it any more.

I am starting to lose it a bit now, I am finding it really hard.

I am feeling OK, but I am on anti-depressants now.

However, the strength of the support offered either way may be variable, and because of this people may become very defensive or angry when they cannot resolve issues. The carer may find that learning new skills for adapting to this distress helps them to deal with it as is demonstrated by the interviewees:

I talked to my Community Psychiatric Nurse and the Alzheimer's Society; they were very good.

Make sure you are passed on to the specialists as quickly as possible and get the help you will need.

We go on coach tours now with friends and that works.

We have very helpful neighbours who take us shopping.

There are no practical problems, I just do everything.

We still managed to go out to friends, but I knew when to stop.

I have applied for a part time post, to give me something interesting to do.

We used to go out for meals a lot, but only occasionally now. I have to plan ahead.

She won't eat in a restaurant but I just have to accept that. You have to learn to deal with it. We can be in toilets for ages, so I just keep shouting out to people that we won't be long.

We laughed about it and that relieved a lot of the frustration a lot of the time.

I feel good just now because he's settled.

I had to realise that if he didn't go I would be the next to be unwell.

I read the Alzheimer's Society leaflet and it reassured me that these things are normal for this illness.

Sometimes it was hard, but I had to remember it was the disease making him behave badly, not him.

It is vital for all involved in this caring situation to understand the implications of such severe stress and the higher risk of developing an abusive relationship (Homer and Gilliard, 1990). We know from this source and from organisational research carried out more recently by Action on Elder Abuse (which is supported by Age Concern England) that there are key factors which influence this risk. They include an increase in dependency, which is inevitable in caring; when the carer has psychological, environmental or other health and social issues which add to the pressure of caring; and when there are difficult behaviours, which is often a problem in people with dementia. As a result of these issues carers do not automatically become abusive, but there is a higher risk of them developing routines and strategies which can become abusive simply by poor care or neglect. Deliberate or active abuse is also heightened in these conditions without adequate support being put in place. There are many policy papers and new laws trying to protect people in these situations, which almost all indicate the need to consider that abuse is possible in any situation and also preventable (Department of Health, 1999; Nursing and Midwifery Council, 2000; Department of Health, 2000, 2001, 2004).

Spirituality

The use of a belief system of some kind is well known to help and support people through difficult times but this does not need to be in the form of a religion. Many people find that just developing a certain perspective about life can also help. The need to understand a person's culture is essential in helping carers to provide meaningful and therapeutic care (Kanitsaki, 2002, pp. 17–27). The understanding of spirituality can be much more aligned to particular belief for an individual and the carer must be able to acknowledge and assist the person with dementia to use their faith if it is something they benefit from. It is simple to forget about a religious belief if the sufferer has also forgotten. Bryden and MacKinlay (2002, pp. 69–75) identify a case of a woman who experiences dementia, and looks at the strategies used by carers to help the woman continue with her faith by feeling God's love through others.

> I am spiritual, but don't go to church. It helps me to see this not as a burden but a learning curve.
>
> A lot of things had become too much, we both used our strong faith to help us through it.
>
> Often when we went to church, even now, he is very settled.

The level of importance attached to spirituality, faith and religion is a key consideration in assisting someone with very distressing problems. The need for them to be supported in maintaining very strong beliefs despite memory complications can be seen as an almost integral part of understanding them and how they want to live their lives. In the older person with dementia or memory loss this aspect of caring may be even more paramount, as it involves the consideration of a possible search for meaning in life, although many young people can be trying to achieve this level of self-introspection as well. Eriksson's 8th stage of life identifies this as 'Integrity vs Despair', and can be used in the examination of life stages (Stuart-Hamilton, 2000). The need of the individual to find meaning in life or not is the issue highlighted here within ageing theories, but is perhaps limited in its very focused approach to age. Spirituality is also an important concept, which can be linked to the feelings around loss of role and meaning and the effect this may have on a person's motivation to continue with life and functioning. Our lives are made up of lots of parts from which we may or may not find spiritual meaning along the way. It must be considered as an aspect of the individual which really never ends as new experiences and feelings will influence it on a daily basis, including experiences of dementia.

The respondents in the interviews were very able to discuss their feelings about how they were coping with the stress, and it became evident that many had similar ideas and issues. These usually focused on uncertainty about the future and the potential need to make a decision about long-term care.

> Just now we are OK, we don't need help, but don't know what will happen in the future.
>
> I think we are OK just now because the carers are here.
>
> At the moment we are coping.
>
> It can be very difficult. I have to look after her tablets as well as mine.

It is easy to assume that the difficult and trying experience of caring is only ever going to be a struggle, but these people tell us that in fact there are ways to cope and that support is actually useful.

> We know who to contact if we need help.
>
> I am sort of coping.
>
> Our neighbours help a lot, we couldn't cope without them.
>
> My brother came and got me to take the tablets (*sufferer*)
>
> Social services told me there is help, just ask.
>
> She goes to the day centre one day and that gives me a break.
>
> It helps when friends and family visit, and I couldn't cope without the day centre and sitting service.
>
> If the support wasn't there I wouldn't be able to cope.
>
> Now in the nursing home he is settled.
>
> Without the Alzheimer's Society support group, my CPN and my husband I couldn't cope.

Adapting the day-to-day routines can often alleviate the stress on carers and, as shown here, many depend on the support they have to do so. The inability to make these changes may lead to carers having to make premature decisions about the care needs of the person and/or becoming too distressed themselves to continue caring effectively.

> She's not going into a nursing home or anything like that while I can still look after her.

> I hope we can carry on as he is for a while. I know he will become more confused and less mobile and will need a lot more care at home, but I will keep him here as long as I can.

> We will get more help if we need it.

> I am going to have to make a decision about long-term care. I want her at home just now though. I want our kids to have our money and not to pay for care. I think it will be when she can't walk, then I may have to.

> If it continues the way it is now, she will have to go into a home.

There are many considerations for a carer when taking decisions about professional care and nursing homes. The concerns around finance are real and can become quite distressing to a couple who feel that their money should not be used for nursing care, which is necessary due to the onset of an illness. However, one of the problems of trying to bring the problems of dementia into society as a social as well as medical problem has contributed to changes in statutory service provision. If we try to move dementia out of the health and disease descriptions and diagnoses categories, then it may be excluded and seen as a social problem only. This is a problem issue when trying to maintain health and support, and the reason why the care of people with dementia has recently moved into the remit of social services. Nursing care is free at the point of delivery in the UK, but the hotel service provided by the nursing home is not, and people often have to pay for this. Social workers and health care teams can advise on local or regional funding.

How we can help ourselves and each other

■ **Understand own stress and learn to identify indicators**: The individual person will adapt to and cope with the variable situations in very different and possibly surprising ways. It is essential to begin trying to see these changes in character as a means of identifying a communications system.

The familiarity developed by a carer with their own feelings and responses can help them to establish patterns, behaviours and general coping levels. The carer can also use this awareness to identify in the person with dementia how their own behaviours affect that of the sufferer. As a result, it may be possible to notice and, if needed, change those behaviours. This can be achieved by the carer spending some time regularly discussing the patterns (daily recording will help with this), with someone who can help them to recognise where things may be going well or when things need to change.

- **Learn to recognise depressive symptoms**: Once it has been established that the carer, and possibly the sufferer, are able to identify their feelings and responses to each other, it may become easier to identify changes to these adaptations in lifestyle as becoming too much too cope with. The list offered earlier in this chapter describes common symptoms of depression and is repeated here for convenience, but it is important to remember that the significance of any of these symptoms depends very much on the individual and whether they have changed to become this way or not.

  - *Emotions*: Sadness, tearfulness, loss of pleasure in usual activities, feeling hopeless and guilty
  - *Motivation*: Increased dependency on others, low energy and fatigue and poor concentration
  - *Cognitive*: Negative expectations and self-image, difficulty making decisions which would have been easy before, preoccupation with illness and any interest expressed in self-harm or suicide
  - *Psychomotor*: Changes in appetite or sleep and consequent weight loss or sleep deprivation, reduced sexual drive and function, early wakening and sleeping day instead of night
  - *Physical*: Changes in body patterns like constipation/diarrhoea, stomach cramps, nausea or irregular menstrual cycles

- **Develop new coping skills**: People are often unaware of the support which is available to them and also sometimes refuse to accept either the need for it or the value of it. As can be seen in the comments, the support offered to carers is vital to maintaining them in a way which means they have some quality of life and can continue to cope. The support can be professional or non-professional, but it is absolutely necessary to anyone in a caring situation. It needs to be accessed, and this may be difficult for anyone who is new to the problems or to using the services. The key thing to remember is that the GP can be the first port of call to get information and direction about where and how to get that support.

- **Identify risk factors in caring relationship**: It is a professional responsibility to be assessing the level of stress at any time, but it is also an ethical concern that formal carers become familiar enough with a family to be able to identify care needs before the risk factors increase. The caring role is one inherent with stress and has potential for abuse; therefore it is essential that all carers are able to discuss concerns regularly and express frustrations. Identifying the risk of abuse involves an awareness of the potential for risk and its transition into reality. The risk management cycle identified by Ryan (1999) helps to clarify a process to go through which involves the identification of potential to harm the self or others and the risk of it actually occurring.

Key elements of any risk assessment in a professional or non-professional context include developing a familiarity with accepted patterns in the relationship and seeing the assessment in perspective. This does not mean, though, that an abusive relationship that has gone on for years, and is causing distress to a person, should not be dealt with now.

The use of established tools of risk measurement for consistency in an open and discursive way with the people involved can only enhance their accuracy in predicting the level of risk.

The safety of the person at risk is a concern for any carer and all action following the identification of the risk should be sensitive and involve action in the best interests of the pair or group involved.

It is always a good idea to record anything unusual: changing behaviours or responses, conversations about concerns, etc.

Always accept a person's identification of being abused, even if not very credible. All feelings are valid and should be dealt with.

- **Develop awareness of spiritual need**: Explore and discuss the key beliefs and values of an individual through the use of general conversation. If communication is limited then the use of interpretation of life stories, previous behaviours and responses to prompts about spiritual, religious or faith beliefs can be used to establish a baseline from which to develop this knowledge.

  Use appropriate support services to provide the kind of spiritual support that has been established as important to the individual: clergy, counselling, discussions around hopes and fears, and the many ethical and value-based decisions made about the individual's life. The use of creative art, emphasising significant faiths in the general environment, combines to ensure the maintenance of spiritual integrity.

This chapter has led into many aspects of the psychological and emotional affects of living with memory loss and dementia. Some general coping skills combined with more specific actions offer professional and non-professional carers a framework from which to base their care strategy, and all need to be developed further within the individual's perspective.

References

Bryden, C. (2005) *Dancing with Dementia. My Story of Living Positively with Dementia*. Jessica Kingsley, London.

Bryden, C. and MacKinlay, E. (2002) Dementia – a spiritual journey. In: *Mental Health and Spirituality in Later Life* (ed. E. MacKinley), pp. 69–75. Haworth Pastoral Press, New York.

Craig, C. and Killick, J. (2004) Reaching out with the arts: meeting with the person with dementia. In: *Dementia and Social Exclusion: Marginalised Groups and Marginalised Areas of Dementia Research, Care and Practice* (eds. A. Innes, C. Archibald and C. Murphy), p. 184. Jessica Kingsley, London.

DSM-IV (*Diagnostic and Statistical Manual of Mental Disorders*, 4th edn) (1994) American Psychiatric Association, Washington.

Department of Health (1999) *No Secrets*. HMSO, London.

Department of Health (2000) *Caring About Carers*. HMSO, London.

Department of Health (2001) *The National Service Framework for Older People*. HMSO, London.

Department of Health (2004) *Who cares? Information and Support for the Carers of People with Dementia*. HMSO, London.

Fine, A. (2002) *The Granny Project*. Egremont Books, UK.

Gilliard, J. (1995) *The Long Winding Road: a Young Person's Guide to Dementia*. Wrightson Biomedical Publishing, UK.

Homer, C. and Gilliard, A. C. (1990) Abuse of elderly people by their carers. *British Medical Journal*, **301**, 1359–62.

ICD-10 (*International Classification of Mental and Behavioural Disorders*, 10th edn) (1992) World Health Organisation, Geneva.

Innes, A., Archibald, C. and Murphy, C. (eds.) (2004) *Dementia and Social Exclusion: Marginalised Groups and Marginalised Areas of Dementia Research, Care and Practice*. Jessica Kingsley, London.

Kanitsaki, O. (2002) Mental health, cultural and spiritual: implications for the effective psychotherapeutic care of Australia's ageing migrant population. In: *Mental Health and Spirituality in Later Life* (ed. E. MacKinley), pp. 17–37. Haworth Pastoral Press, New York.

Kitwood, T. (1997) *Dementia Reconsidered. The Person Comes First*. Open University Press, Maidenhead.

MacKinlay, E. (ed.) (2002) *Mental Health and Spirituality in Later Life*. Haworth Pastoral Press, New York.

Mental Health Act 1983 Review (summary) (2000). HMSO, London.

Mental Health Foundation (2005) *The Milk's in the Oven.* http://www.mental-health.org.uk/.

Miller, S. (2003) *The Story of My Father.* Bloomsbury, London.

National Institute for Aging (2002) *Caregiver Guide: Tips for Caregivers of People with Alzheimer's Disease.* National Institute for Aging, US Department of Health and Human Services Public health service, Publication no. 01-4013.

Nay, R. (2003) *Sexuality and the Older Person.* Unpublished PhD Dissertation, La Trobe University, Australian Centre for Evidence-Based Aged Care.

Norman, I. and Ryrie, I. (2004) *The Art and Science of Mental Health Nursing: A Textbook of Principles and Practice.* Open University Press, New York, pp. 572–3.

Nursing and Midwifery Council (2000) *Code of Professional Conduct.* Nursing and Midwifery Council, London.

Office for National Statistics (2000) *Psychiatric Morbidity among Adults Living in Private Households, 2000.* http://www.statistics.gov.uk/downloads/theme_health/psychmorb.pdf.

Office for National Statistics (2003) *The Mental Health of Older People.* HMSO, London

Ryan, T. (1999) *Managing Crisis and Risk in Mental Health Nursing.* Stanley Thornes, Cheltenham.

Shriver, M. (2004) *What's Happening to Grandpa?* Little, Brown and Co./ Warner Books, London.

Stuart-Hamilton, I. (2000) *The Psychology of Ageing: an Introduction*, 3rd edn. Jessica Kingsley, London.

World Health Organization (2006) *Department of Reproductive Health and Research.* http://www.who.int/reproductive-health/gender/sexual-health/.

Zarit, S., Orr, J. and Zarit, J. M. (1987) *The Hidden Victims of Alzheimer's Disease.* New York University Press, New York.

CHAPTER 6

Support in a caring situation

Learning points on the need for support:

■ Getting a diagnosis, and how this event can be more accessible and supportive
■ What to do when caring, including using services, technology and medication
■ How we can help ourselves and each other by learning about the different
supports available and how to access them

Support is an essential part of caring, professional or non-professional. The type
of support that is useful to different people is as individual as the problems they
face on a day-to-day basis.

The interviews considered this issue in a practical way and can offer
examples of how people found support, how to use it to its best effect and
how to adapt it to their own needs. The main categories in this section deal
with before and after diagnosis, practical advice on coping with caring roles
using the support, and what statutory support services are actually available
to people.

Keady *et al.* (2003) identified through research key areas which were important to people involved in caring and being cared for. These findings are promoted in the book as a structure of themes that can be considered by professionals to help provide support in the home. They include emotional support and
counselling, diagnostic support, dealing with threats to autonomy, maintaining
the status quo, dealing with critical incidents and providing access to services.
The concerns expressed by this group of respondents focus very much on the
issues that concern them on a daily basis and are not prioritised by the availability of services or professionals. A less useful approach of the sufferer and
informal carer just accepting what they are given and having to try to fit into an
inflexible support service is unacceptable.

The current advancement in caring is based on the needs being met by the
adapting service and the individuals being cared for, rather than the illness, and
is advocated here.

Our group had similar concerns and feelings and most support services that
were found to be useful were those that can, or at least try to, be flexible in their
approach.

Diagnosis

A major problem in accessing help is the general lack of awareness of its availability or need. Many people struggle with the symptoms of memory loss and potentially dementia for up to 36 months before they even go to the GP (Heymanson, 2005).

It is important therefore for health and social care professionals to work alongside voluntary organisations or support groups in the community to ensure that when people do face these challenges they have a point of contact which can, at the very least, direct them to the appropriate help.

However, despite these organisations' attempts at health promotion events, such as National Alzheimer's Week in September and information distribution in GP surgeries, it is still impossible for everyone to be aware of everything that may or may not affect them in the future. It is therefore relied upon that most people will eventually think to go to the GP and can then be directed into the support network based on an appropriate assessment.

This means that the initial consultation by the GP, practice nurse or social carer must be acute and immediately supportive. Any other response can have the potential effect of driving people away from the very source of help they need.

> We felt there was nothing wrong and she was just being awkward. We eventually went to the doctor and she was referred for an assessment, but it was delayed as we were in a different area from her home address.

> It was devastating 'cause we really thought he hadn't got it, I was on my own.

> We went to the GP and she had lost weight, down to 6 st 13 lb. When she went to get the diagnosis from a neurologist he was shouting at her for not following his instructions. He just told us it was Alzheimer's and she started crying, saying she was too young. He was very abrasive.

Despite these extreme and evidently distressing experiences there are also comments which determine the effectiveness of a more compassionate approach to people who are being given a diagnosis.

> I talked about it to my CPN and Alzheimer's Society; they were very good.

> The GP sent him to Millbrook mental health unit right away and he was diagnosed straight away. I knew it would be dementia and I felt some relief that it wasn't my imagination.

He did prescribe Aricept and got her a private prescription and put us in touch with Alzheimer's Society. They got her referred to a consultant psychiatrist; he came very quickly and helped.

The professionals involved in these situations do not by any means represent the overall response in health and social care services. These do demonstrate a negative response by the services and put a lot more strain on an already increasingly difficult situation, whilst a supportive approach from the beginning helps to alleviate the stress.

How we can help ourselves and each other

- **Professionals develop awareness of dementia and memory loss**: In the current agenda of inter-professional training and working it is possible to see a future where this problem of ignorance of dementia and its effect on people's lives can be minimised significantly. The creation of new roles like liaison staff between specialities and consultant-type care staff will lead to a wider understanding of the need for health promotion strategies in the community and can only enhance the general public awareness. There is no need for people to become specialists in every aspect of their health, but they do need to know where to go for help when they have problems.
- **Go to the person you trust most**: The potential carer has to make decisions about who to turn to for guidance, how to overcome the fear they have themselves as well as that of the sufferer, and of the consequences of any decisions. The decision to seek help itself will not incur consequences, only answers to questions. The person with memory loss may need some support, but not a lot, at first, or they may need crisis support. This all depends on the situation, but the decisions about care are all up to the person themselves and the carer, by legal right of determination. The recent passing of the Capacity to Consent Act 2005 means that all people assessed by any professional must be assumed to have capacity to consent unless proven otherwise. This new law will not be in force until 2007, but its impact is significant in ensuring that the individual's personal choices are not overtaken by professional judgement. The relationship that is formed between the professionals, sufferers and carers depends very much on a trusting, balanced approach, and this goes both ways. It is vital for people with dementia and carers to establish a level of trust with the professionals so that decisions can be made based on experience, evidence and the best interests of those involved.

What to do when caring

People lose skills as a matter of course when dementia progresses. The assumption that any loss of skill, to any degree, means a lost ability in everything can be misleading and ultimately detrimental to the sufferer's ability to retain skills of independence. The nature of the problems means that a person's ability to manage day-to-day tasks is affected by an inability to remember how to do it or a lack of concentration on the task, or just simply forgetting that it needs to be done. These problems can lead to issues of safety and the potential for the person's health and social ability to deteriorate if they forget to eat, go to the toilet or lock the door, get lost or generally become unable to maintain their previous life skills.

> She can't cook or anything like that, she couldn't go further than the end of the street on her own.
>
> We do everything for him. He can't do anything.
>
> I do all the cooking and cleaning, and our daughters help. She would leave the gas on and stuff.
>
> She has lost interest in any jobs, although I have tried to involve her.
>
> He does nothing in the house. He used to do all the fixing and DIY and now he just says it doesn't need doing.

Despite these concerns it is possible to maintain a level of independence for the sufferer by seeing these tasks in a way that breaks them down into more realistic and resolvable activities.

> I kept trying to get him to sit at the table, as he ate himself when sat down.
>
> She still eats herself but can't recognise the cutlery and needs help.
>
> Over the last two weeks his speech, understanding, awareness and alertness are much better. The medical profession are very surprised and can't explain it; just now he will understand if you speak slowly. I feel good just now because he is settled, although I know it won't last forever.

The person with dementia may still be able to voice feelings about still being able to do tasks, and it is important to try to establish this to prevent frustration and distress at this time and later through other means of communication.

> I still feel I ought to be doing it, but can't (*sufferer*)

The ability of the carer to see these skills as retainable in some ways will help them to prevent a false dependence. The carer can encourage continued involvement in day-to-day tasks with help, support or supervision as is necessary. However, it is also very tempting to ensure that safety is maintained, jobs are done properly and that they can get out of the door on time for an appointment by doing it themselves.

He does what I tell him.

I spend the night checking on her.

I dress her and she mostly lets me.

The statutory (government) support networks

The statutory services consist of many variations around the country and it is vital to find out what is available in the local area. There are many core services which are consistent, but generally there will be differences across all areas regarding what is available and when. Some of the support services that can be useful are seen in the following quotations:

We go to the memory clinic every 6 months.

We had an assessment and were to get hand rails on the stairs but they didn't fit. Did get a seat for the bath which does help.

We go to a monthly support group with Alzheimer's Society. That gives us people who have the same problems to talk to.

We are just waiting for Age Concern to come and talk to us about finances.

We got a CPN and they told us about Alzheimer's Society.

Somebody else put us on to the Alzheimer's Society.

He went to MIND. We had a sitting service and he had respite two weeks out of the month, although that meant he was out of his routine when he returned. It was for about 10 years; then it got too much.

Social services and the doctor assessed him and he went into a nursing home.

He went to a day centre and he enjoyed it, so he goes two days a week.

After the diagnosis, a CPN started visiting and a social worker assessed her. After a few months, though, she had to come and live with us.

I saw an advert in the local paper for Alzheimer's Society and contacted them. They really helped me. She gave me information sheets and the meetings are very good. I gave the leaflets to people in the family.

She started a day centre and seems to enjoy it.

The list of organisations at the end of this chapter may help the carer to locate the different support in their area independently, but the statutory services will always be able to help people access this support.

Technology as a support

Technology is an ever-expanding area in dementia care and offers enormous potential for support, now and in the future. At present it is still very experimental, other than in basic systems like door alarms, timer switches on cookers and barometer-controlled heating. When asked about the use of technology to help with problems of dementia and caring most of the respondents found it hard to imagine what kind of devices might help them, and few had even heard of the concept.

An alarm on the front door might help with him leaving the front door open.

Alarms and gadgets only helped so much.

Things that would help me are not technological, because our house and the area is quite safe.

Some of the emerging technologies can be seen in experimental environments like the Bristol Smart House, Housing 21, and the new development in Scotland of a complex of smart houses (Alzheimer's Scotland/Cube Housing, 2005). The Scottish example demonstrates how technology can be used to help people maintain a level of independence with as little risk as possible. The housing development is a small complex of self-contained flats. They are designed to be dementia-friendly and to help develop a community amongst the residents. They are set out in open plan to avoid confusion and residents can see the whole length of the flat to help them find where they are going. In the kitchen there are see-through cupboards which assist in identifying food and its whereabouts. Colour psychology has been used to guard against getting lost, and lighting is uniform to prevent disorientating and distressing shadows appearing. The sen-

Some assistive technologies

■ Machine learning techniques. This is a self-automated system that will learn a person's pattern of daily movement and activity, detect abnormal changes early and cue activity.

■ 'Auto-minder' models, updates and maintains the individual's plans. Maintains a memory of that performance and is able to reason about which reminders to issue and when.

■ 'Telemedicine' is specific to people who love alone. It has been suggested that people with dementia who live alone have less functional impairment, and therefore this automated system of reminding may be manageable.

■ 'Solo' is about helping people by instructing them how to carry out an activity rather than just when to do it.

■ 'GPS for people with cognitive disability' is the use of satellite navigation to help those at risk of getting lost. If a person gets lost it will tell them what to do to find the way and overcome errors when disorientated.

sory garden for stimulation is self-contained and helps people to return easily to the house. The use of motion detectors helps staff to monitor whereabouts and safety without being too intrusive.

Many technologies are currently being developed and the Alzheimer's Society International demonstrated some of these at the 9th International conference in 2004 (see box).

There are of course many issues with this emerging technology, despite its obvious potential to help people live more independent lives. The possibility of technical failure and the person being unaware or unable to deal with the action required to get assistance to repair it needs to be overcome. The emotional distress caused to people when trying to carry out simple tasks is written about regularly and the use of a very foreign-looking object like a handheld computer may inspire the same anxieties. Also, the issues of privacy and some very intrusive and covert monitoring technology have to be considered in terms of the ethical questions raised. The person involved may not be aware of being monitored, and whilst it seems a great way of maintaining independence it may also be a means of further eroding their basic human rights to privacy and self-determination.

The lack of these technologies except in special projects is partly because of the newness of the idea, but also because of the cost. Who will pay for such expensive means of support? The cost of health and social care is already limited to certain criteria which usually relate to maintenance of safety, security and health risks. They do not often extend to quality of life needs, such as just making life with memory problems or dementia easier. These technologies are expensive and each has specific uses which limits its application to everyone and bulk buying. However, it may be that the use of them in day centres, for example, is a way of using them efficiently until these problems are overcome. The assumption that a technological gadget will help everyone is just the same as the idea that all approaches to care will help everyone and just as destructive, but a lot more expensive.

People with sensory problems such as poor hearing, sight or mobility may have problems with using the technology those who are isolated, living alone, poverty-stricken and homeless have no access to such means. People in different generations will have different expectations and abilities because of life experience, and this will ensure that the use of these support means will be ever changing. The questions that further research into this area must consider involve whether technology can indeed improve people's quality of life, safety and security and whether it can be adapted to the many variations of individuals' lives.

Lastly on this point, it is important to acknowledge the potential invasive nature of this kind of development for a group of people who are vulnerable to abuse. It must be considered always that these are human beings who naturally need human contact and support and the replacement of that with technology in the extreme is a real concern to take seriously. This development can be paralleled with 'task-orientated care', which tries to get the job done regardless of any loss of individuality. Perhaps a compromise could involve the use of technology for functional problems and behaviours, while the emotional and attachment support continues to be offered by human contact. Just because we can do something does not mean that we should just do it without careful ethical consideration.

Medication as a support

Medication can serve as a support when used appropriately. Most people's experience with it may be fraught with worry and anxiety, but essentially it does have a place in helping individuals to feel and cope better.

> She got depressed when it started when she knew something was wrong, she had no treatment for that.

> GP put her on some anti-depressants, side effects meant they had to change to a different one.

He did start to get a bit depressed and was staring at the wall. The CPN came, then spoke to the doctor and they doubled the anti-depressant and that helped.

She was started on anti-depressants and her Aricept reduced. They helped her to calm down a lot. It really lifted her spirits.

He had anti-depressants which helped him when he was crying all the time. He also had some to calm him down and help him sleep, and those worked OK, no side effects.

The doctor refused to give her sleeping tablets. She had something to help her calm down, but they just made her drowsy and sleepy all the time. I stopped it.

They didn't put him on anti-depressants, but his meds for his water works have an anti-depressant action and that seems to have lifted his mood a bit.

The worries that people have about medication are real and should be taken seriously by professionals whilst still trying to ensure that people with dementia and carers are aware of the benefits when it is appropriate. The use of medication in this area of care is fraught with complications. Often the person is older and the natural ageing process makes people more vulnerable to the negative effects of medications. All prescriptions given out are done so by professionals who are well aware of the evidence that suggests these vulnerabilities, and they take this responsibility very seriously. However, problems can occur, depending on individual tolerance, compliance, and awareness of looking out for side effects.

Medication has also become quite specialist recently in helping people with the problems of dementia. The drugs which are used mostly in this group of people are called acetylcholinesterase inhibitors. The action of these drugs assumes that a neurotransmitter, acetylcholine, is being broken down too quickly by an enzyme in the brain of a person with dementia, whose levels of acetylcholine are already low. Therefore these drugs inhibit the enzyme from carrying this out, potentially allowing the normal process of acetylcholine production and improving brain function. Commonly known as Aricept, Exelon, Ebixa, Memantine etc., these medications have provided people with some hope of medical progress in the battle to deal more effectively with dementia.

It is important to remember that these drugs have an effect on the symptoms, but do not cure the illness, nor do they claim to. Some research has demonstrated that there are some clear benefits to this medication if given to the right people at the right time of the illness. These benefits include increased concentration, general alertness and even improvement in skills. However, some research has also suggested that they have little effect. This could suggest that the effect is dependent on a psychological reaction or that it is being prescribed to the wrong people. Continued research is assessing the effectiveness of prevention with more natural sources of anti-oxidants: vitamin E and ginkgo biloba. Also considered in research are alternative approaches, such as reducing inflammation in the brain with non-steroidal anti-inflammatory drugs used for strokes etc., and the effects of the different drugs for degrees of severity and types of dementia. This means that, as with all aspects of treatment and care, one drug does not fit all. Prescription must be based on individual need, and medical research continues to develop this field while doctors continue to evaluate its use. Recent changes in UK research into the efficacy of drugs have seen the development of the National Institute for Clinical Excellence (NICE), and they are responsible for the decision to make certain anti-dementia drugs available to certain people through NHS prescriptions. The criteria for each person are assessed at a memory clinic and the effects monitored.

> She has been on Aricept for three years, don't know if it's worked because we don't know what she'd be like without it. No side effects or problems though.

> She started on Aricept, which was good, then that had to be changed to Reminyl. Also Ebixa and that's not helping, she's become a bit nasty.

> I had to fight for Aricept as they hadn't given a diagnosis. They eventually gave him it and he was better at thinking and could do things methodically. But it made him tired and not wanting to do very much.

> He got Aricept but that was changed to Ebixa. I don't think it is as good.

> He tried Aricept but had terrible side effects and that was stopped.

How we can help ourselves and each other

■ **Promote independence**: As discussed before, the promotion of independence can benefit all involved in the long run, as it means that skills are not inevitably lost and can often be maintained. This maintained level of skill can mean that carers have less to do, a welcome relief from the constant pressure of meeting needs. It is also necessary to remain realistic with this aspiration and ensure that an appropriate level of guidance is still available and that tasks or activities are adapted to what the sufferer can do. The insistence on maintaining shaving skills in a man may have to be adapted to using an electric shaver to ensure safety; the washing of dishes can be done together to ensure that they are done properly; and the business of going to the toilet could be done by prompting rather than taking.

- **Find support and services**: The NHS and social care facilities are immense in the UK and are there to be used. The problems that occur within them and which are commonly reported by anecdote can be a little misleading. Generally, people find the main support they need from this resource. Access it as soon as concerns are raised to ensure that time is not lost in getting help.

  The other support services, such as voluntary organisations and support groups, are also a vital lifeline in this experience. Use the list at the end of the chapter to begin sifting through these and finding out where and what is available locally.

- **Become familiar with technology**: Currently the resources of technology are not readily available to the general public, as many are still under development and those that are available are very expensive. It is useful for campaigning and future reference to be aware of what is being introduced and being able to decipher its potential impact on people's lives.

- **Explore possibilities with prescribed medication**: Accepting the potential need for medication will mean that if it is suggested carers will be prepared and able to question its necessity and monitor its effect on the individual accurately. Learn about types of medication, including anti-depressants and the anti-dementia drugs in general. Find out about the potential side effects of specific drugs when prescribed so that monitoring is more accurate and reporting back to medical staff is more effective.

Statutory services in the UK

Learning points on the local and national care offered by the NHS and social services

- Statutory services in the UK and their relevance to people with care needs
- Specific issues of younger people with dementia
- How we can help ourselves and each other by gaining information

It is possible to travel the length of the UK and find many variations in care approaches and services available to people with memory problems and dementia and their carers. This does not mean that there is no consistency, but could be explained by the very basis of using services for individual need and local concerns for application.

The main statutory services are constructed based on UK law, and are then adapted to work in particular areas of the country. The most recent addition to this – the Capacity to Consent Act 2005 – is applicable everywhere, but it will need to be applied according to need in a particular situation. The combination of health and social care is a UK-wide strategy instituted by the Health Act 1999 and Health and Social Care Act 2001, but its use can be seen in different ways by adaptations to services based on resources and need.

Working together

As a result of these developments there has been much progress in dementia care services and their alliances, commonly known in professional circles as collaborative care. These involve professionals, carers, people with dementia, voluntary organisations and educational approaches all trying to work together to establish a more consistent and effective service for all.

Many of the respondents identify the problems which are meant to be overcome by collaborative care:

> She was admitted into hospital for assessment. She was not looked after and we brought her home against medical advice.

> We had respite two weeks out of four, but it meant he had lost his routine when he got back.

It is evident in these comments that sometimes the support offered by the services is of limited use. This kind of problem is one which should be addressed by professionals as real when discussing care options with individuals to ensure that anxieties about the changes in quality of care are considered and that those areas which continue to provide poor standards of care can be avoided.

The combination of services is now commonplace in statutory service provision and is mentioned as a matter of course by the people interviewed. Collaborative care is in place; the only question is whether it is working and how it can be developed.

> Got a CPN and went to support group.

> He went to MIND and we had a sitting service and respite.

> He did put us in touch with the Alzheimer's Society and they got her assessed by a consultant psychiatrist.

> After the diagnosis a CPN and social worker assessed her.

Some of the concerns shared by many people living with dementia and its effects are about the legalities of care and finance.

> He was sectioned and I felt I had no choice. [*This means that he was kept in hospital legally, but against his will.*]

> They sectioned him because he was not orientated, but I told them he had been that way for over a year.

> I made a complaint to the hospital, I was so angry about her care. I was offered respite in Newark instead, but it's too far away.

> They stopped the day centre when he had his stroke, 'cause then they couldn't cope with his behaviour.

> I think the professionals should listen to the carers more about whether the person will be better at home or not. I really had to fight with them to have him at home; only the CPN and Alzheimer's Society agreed with me. They all agreed later it was the right decision.

The professional assessment may well conflict with the carer's individual perspective as a result of resources or fundamental beliefs about the cause of a particular issue. Professionals base their knowledge on evidence from research as well as the individual experience, and they are, and should be, accountable for decisions they make or advice that they offer. Resources are also based on statistical need rather than individual need and therefore can be very rigid and uncompromising, but with the interests of the general public as a whole at their basis. Informal carers, however, can have limited knowledge of this evidence, if at all, and their only priority is for the welfare of the individuals concerned. The resulting conflicting priorities and concerns can lead to a breakdown in relationships which are essentially meant to be supportive.

Examples of collaborative partnerships include the changes in health teams to include many different professionals working together in one organisation (or building) and seeing clients as a team. Therefore a mental health team may consist of a nurse, social worker, occupational therapist and psychiatrist, in consultation with voluntary organisations in their normal practices. Changes in the funding and structural arrangements of these organisations to accommodate this are complex, but are in place as a result of legislation like the Health and Social Care Act and the National Service Frameworks. A person referred to the statutory services will be seen by a member of the team, and for true collaboration to work this person and carers will become part of the team and devise the plan of care together.

Younger people and dementia

'There are not many places for young people with dementia' indicates the general consensus in the dementia care field that this is indeed an under-resourced area. The needs of younger people as a group may involve many different issues, such as continued occupation, continued physical ability and family responsibilities.

> He was working, then he went off sick. Redundancy was threatened so he went back. Then after six months he broke down: he couldn't travel on the bus, was getting paranoid about people talking about him. Then he got early retirement on sick grounds, which he didn't want, but accepted that he would have a better quality of life.

> How would we cope, as I am disabled too?

> She started making mistakes at work and her employers were concerned about her.

> She stopped work after she broke down in tears and they sent her home.

The development of collaborative care has provided a means of trying to share the costs of providing a service to a statistically small number of people by combining resources and ensuring that younger people are not assumed to have the same issues as each other, or indeed of older people. The case for individuality is not only an ethical concern, but one of finance also.

Despite these problems it is easy to see examples of effective support and how the statutory services and organisations can and do offer very supportive relationships.

> The Alzheimer's Society helps with advice about forms and benefits and meetings, someone else who understands.

> We had rails and a shower put in, that helps us both. She goes to a day centre once a week and that gives me a break.

> We used respite twice before and it went well.

> What I have now is good.

> His pattern changes after respite, so we don't know what he'll be like. I have managed to get him the same carers when he goes into respite, and that has helped a lot with maintaining his routine and calming him when he is on the ward.

Keeping to structures of the day like day centres puts a lot of stress on me to get him ready. I changed how I talked to him: now I say someone is coming to see you rather than fetch you.

She is as glad to go to the day centre as I am to have a break.

He is settled in the nursing home. I know this because he is not agitated when I go to see him. I think the quality of our relationship is as improved as it could be because we can just enjoy each other without the pressures.

He goes to the day centre and is always pleased to see me when I collect him.

How we can help ourselves and each other

- **Become familiar with UK law on care**: The laws and regulations are very confusing, but this text and others like it offer a way of finding out the basics about individuals' rights under the law, including the Mental Health Act 1983, Human Rights Act 1998 and the Capacity to Consent Act 2005. These rights are generalisable and apply to every person in the country, but it is necessary to get appropriate advice on what they mean for the individual. The organisations listed at the end of this chapter can help to decipher these issues and those of a financial nature in an understandable and useful way.

  The localised resources can vary, but just getting advice from these organisations will decipher the individual's needs and bring it together with the local resource available.
- **Develop knowledge of care issues**: Textbooks and specialist care books can often be difficult to understand for non-professionals, but there are many resources provided by these organisations, as well as books like this which can offer guidance at the level that is appropriate. Knowing about the problems encountered by people in these situations and how to cope with them is essential. Sufferers and carers alike need to know what they are dealing with, and what their options and rights are, to be able to make informed decisions. Use of more advanced reading in books and journals can enhance that ability by helping people to consider not just the facts of the situation but the ever-changing and developing debates around ethics, care strategies and policies.

References

Alzheimer's Scotland/Cube Housing (2005) New development opens in Glasgow. *Journal of Dementia Care*, **13**(5), news item.

Alzheimer's Society (2004) *9th International Conference on Alzheimer's Disease and Related Disorders*. Philadelphia.

Carnwell, R. and Buchanan, J. (2005) *Effective Practice in Health and Social Care: a Partnership Approach*. Open University Press, Berkshire.

Heymanson, C. (2005) Help before diagnosis. *Journal of Dementia Care*, **13**(5), 17.

Keady, J., Clarke, C. L. and Adams, T. (2003) *Community Mental Health Nursing and Dementia Care: Practice Perspectives*. Open University Press, Maidenhead.

Resource information and organisations

Age Concern
Astral House
1268 London Road
London
SW16 4ER

Tel: 020 8765 7200
http://www.ageconcern.org.uk/
Helpline: 0800 009966

Age Concern Cymru
4th Floor
1 Cathedral Road
Cardiff
CF11 9SD

Tel: 02920 371566
http://www.accymru.org.uk/

Age Concern Northern Ireland
3 Lower Crescent
Belfast
BT7 1NR

Tel: 02890 245729
http://www.ageconcernni.org/

Age Concern Scotland
113 Rose Street
Edinburgh
EH2 3DT

Tel: 0131 220 3345
http://www.ageconcernscotland.org.uk/

Alzheimer Scotland
23 Drumsheugh Gardens
Edinburgh
EH3 7RN

Tel: 0131 243 1453
http://www.alzscot.org/
Helpline: 0808 808 3000

The Alzheimer's Society
Gordon House
10 Greencoat Place
London
SW1P 1PH

Tel: 020 7306 0606
http://www.alzheimers.org/
Helpline: 0845 300 0336

Carers UK
20–25 Glasshouse Yard
London
EC1A 4JT

Tel: 020 7490 8818
http://www.carersuk.org/
Tel: 0808 808 7777

Caring Matters
132 Gloucester Place
London
NW1 6DT

Tel: 020 7402 2702
http://www.caring-matters.org.uk/

Citizens Advice Bureau
Myddleton House
115–123 Pentonville Road
London
N1 9LZ
Tel: 020 7833 2181

http://www.adviceguide.org.uk/

Crossroads Care Schemes
10 Regent Place
Rugby
Warwickshire
CV21 2PN

Tel: 01788 573653
http://www.crossroads.org.uk/

For Dementia
6 Camden High Street
London
NW1 0SH

Tel: 020 7241 8555
http://www.fordementia.org.uk/

Housing 21
Bristol/Gloucester Smart House
Longwood House
Love Lane
Cirencester
Gloucester
GL7 1YG

Tel: 01285 659928
http://housing21.co.uk/

MIND
15–19 Broadway
London
E15 4BQ

Tel: 020 8519 2122
Fax: 020 8522 1725
Helpline: 0845 766 0163
http://www.mind.org.uk/

Samaritans
Chris
P.O. Box 90
Stirling
FK8 2SA

Tel: 08457 90 90 90
http://www.samaritans.org/

CHAPTER 7

Coping with daily activities

Grealy *et al.* (2005) discuss many very practical approaches to care. Their underlying philosophy asserts that quality care of people with dementia is created by the carer's ability to develop an awareness of unmet need. They argue that the reduction of 'resistance to care' is a key aspect in ensuring that these needs are met and that resistance in the form of refusal to participate, aggression or hostility on intervention can be overcome by understanding and the appropriate approach. Archibald (2003) also offers practical advice and guidance in care learning. The fundamental beliefs of this strategy are based on the need to see the individual, find pathways through each experience with the person and ensure that individuality is maintained.

Loss of ability

Learning points on the issues of daily routines and adaptations:

- Identifying loss of ability through health promotion and awareness of general support services
- Considering specific areas of ability changing, including household tasks
- How we can help ourselves and each other by accepting frustrations and managing risks

In the early stages of dementia it is very difficult to decide if the problems encountered are part of an early illness or something else. Sometimes it is difficult for individuals to notice the differences in behaviour, as they are not with the person all the time. The person with early symptoms may be very scared and worried, or just not able to recall the difficulties they are having. This results in the family or friends not really finding the truth until things have progressed significantly. Most of the respondents in these interviews said that it was between six months and a year of them first noticing something to them actually accepting that they needed to do something about it. Many people just continue with their lives, either unaware or denying that there is a change in this person.

The people involved, therefore, are never able to access help in early stages because they are not aware of the progression. This presents a dilemma in that this is a crucial point in time for the sufferer to receive assessment and treatment and for both the carer and sufferer to gain access to support. It is hard to see how this problem can be overcome simply because of the need to first identify it by non-professionals. As discussed in Chapter 2, it is clear that there are high-risk groups of people identified. However, these are people from a vast age, social and environmental range and could never be defined in such a way as to find them before the onset of symptoms. Apart from the problem of doing so in practice, there are concerns about invasion of privacy, consent and general scaremongering.

Despite all this, it is possible to continue to cast a general health promotion-type education about dementia which can help the general public to become more aware of tell-tale signs and then how to access advice. The Alzheimer's Society holds a dementia awareness week in September each year, and local health and social care services often try to promote their services generally through GP surgeries and health centres.

The people in the interviews talked about the early symptoms with distress. This seemed to be due to bewilderment and a feeling of loss of control. Many felt that they had little choice in how to deal with the problems and found it difficult to identify them as anything more than just changing personalities.

We went on hols and on the way back he got completely lost when driving home. He got so upset and frustrated. I could remember some of the way but I had to let him do it because he was so upset.

Her driving got erratic.

She got confused about usual stuff and forgot things. She gave a woman in a shop her purse to take the money out. She stopped doing the shopping properly.

Forgetting people, time and places, it just gradually got worse.

She started coming back from the shops having forgotten, not able to remember names of people she met.

Losing his keys, unable to sleep, to cope with life in general.

Forgetting was the first thing and I didn't get out much. (sufferer)

Things needed doing and he just wouldn't do them.

He started saying he couldn't keep up at work, his colleagues at work were phoning me and telling me he wasn't coping.

He has a love of music and used to make sound tapes in his studio upstairs, but then he just couldn't do it.

She didn't really get lost; a few times wandered away in town, but not far. Now she doesn't leave the house without me.

He told me once he couldn't tell the time.

He would try to go out at night saying he wanted to go home. I could usually persuade him not to. During the day he would go out, but I got him to wear an identity bracelet.

It came in stages. One thing would die down then another thing would start. He always made me tea, and then it turned into a cup of water and eventually he made my son a cup of vinegar one night.

He was crying a lot.

Mum used to wander out a lot when she was still at home on her own, and on one occasion the police brought her back as she was nearly knocked over on the new bypass. I had left my number in the house.

She wasn't eating and lost loads of weight. She said she was eating and yet all the shopping was still in the fridge. Said she was going to local café but turned up at the wrong times.

We fell out a lot then, because I didn't know. I'd leave her clean clothes out but she didn't put them on and dried herself with toilet paper.

The police said it was so serious, so I packed her up and took her to my house and she stayed.

The more severe and potentially dangerous or risky the behaviours, the more worried each became. As can be seen, the beginning of symptoms seemed to deteriorate into worrying concerns as time progressed. The changes and behaviours will be discussed now generally as occurring at all stages of the illness.

Household activities

As can be seen, many people have early problems with household tasks which ultimately lead to the initial consultation with a doctor by a very frustrated and worried person or persons.

Some of the problems identified here are involve safety and security, general loss of normal activity and the very obvious change in response to activities which were once commonplace to the individual.

If I go out for a short time I just lock the door.

She lost interest in any jobs although I tried to involve her before.

I do all the cooking; she would leave the gas on.

We get up early, have breakfast and then the day depends on day centre or visits.

I get up and sorted and it takes about two hours to get him up and ready. Go out around lunchtime, have lunch out and in the afternoon go for a walk. Then I may give him a few jobs to do, like weeding or scrubbing the bench.

He goes for a few walks a day and this usually keeps him calm.

He always complies with the patterns or structures I plan, as long as we are going out. He does get a bit frustrated by times and stuff.

We have to change the pattern daily because she is different every day.

I put the washing away and she moves it all when tidying.

Often I just let him do the dishes when he wanted to keep him occupied.

Also demonstrated in the comments are examples of how to cope with these changes, and the key point is concerns adapting the lifestyle. The carer may have to adapt the household chores and tasks. Often this presents problems for those whose routine is based on a long history of defined roles, and the need to learn new skills is often a resented aspect of learning to care. The typical example is shown by the carer who has to take over the cooking. Having never previously cooked, this is a huge undertaking and often quite daunting. Shopping, cleaning, household repairs and gardening are also areas that are often well demarcated between two people before the onset of any problems.

How we can help ourselves and each other

■ **Acceptance of the changes in behaviour and patterns**: If the carer can accept the problems that the person with dementia faces in terms of coping emotionally and practically with a loss of life skills, then they may be able to see that usually there is a way to support and ultimately improve the person's situation and therefore behaviour. Many carers express exasperation about changed behaviours, but assume that it is just the illness that causes them. It may help them to adapt to the changes more effectively to understand that actually, it is not the illness but the individual sufferer's reaction to a very distressing and frightening turn of events in their lives. They need also to accept that sometimes the behaviours are those of a person who has always behaved in that way and that the change of reaction is with the carer.

In this instance it is important to be cautious about the response to prevent any subconscious retaliation.

In household tasks it may be useful to carers to use statutory services like a home help, who could assist with cleaning, and meals on wheels to reduce the amount of cooking needed. The local resource for this kind of service is one which varies but essentially the health/social care professional involved will be able to direct people to what is available. The main point in this aspect of care is the ability to adapt previous patterns and therefore prevent the loss of ability from becoming a source of conflict and distress.

■ **Understand that risk is normal**: Everybody faces risk during the course of a day. People with dementia are not exempt from this. They are also potentially more at risk because of things like disorientation and getting lost, forgetting and leaving the gas on or the front door unlocked, or eating food which is uncooked or past its sell by date. It is obvious that risk factors of safety are increased when a person has these types of problem. It is necessary for carers to be able to assess this risk and minimise it as much as possible. It is, for example, easy to get meals on wheels delivered to prevent eating undercooked food; to remove gas-fired appliances and replace them with electric ones; to or put alarms on doors and reminders etc. around the house, as was demonstrated by the discussion on assistive technologies. All of these measures can minimise the risk of harm to a person with memory problems or dementia. The ability to accept that some risk remains is scary for carers and is often the reason for the imposition of rules, regulations and patterns which inhibit the individual's activity. For example, in a care institution it is very common to find that sufferers are not allowed in the kitchen, as a means of maintaining their safety and the health and hygiene of everyone. It is possible to see the logic in this kind of rule for some, but many people enjoy cooking and this could be a source of therapeutic or just simply enjoyable activity that they could maintain. This small adaptation in regulation could be the difference between an individual's mood changing for the better or worse.

Personal care

Learning points on the changes in ability on a day-to-day basis:

■ Considering self-care and hygiene and the problems of dependence on carers
■ How we can help ourselves and each other by changing perceptions and expectations and prioritising need

■ Sleep, going to the toilet, eating and drinking, medication with food, maintaining skin condition, assessing for pain and changes in social lives all need acknowledging; developing adapting routines and understanding the changes

■ How we can help ourselves and each other by using support services, adapting routines and accepting changes in expectations

Another area seriously affected by forgetfulness and disorientation is a person's ability to maintain their own personal hygiene and care. The changes in this aspect of behaviour are often the most difficult to hide. People notice a previously well-shaven and clean-clothed man who has become dishevelled and apparently untidy. The concern here for professionals is that they do not know the previous patterns of an individual's personal presentation. It is important to remember that one person's unclean and untidy is another's normal practice. The individual also has to cope with either the identification, and the consequent embarrassment of being told, that they are untidy or that they have a body odour. The self-esteem of the individual can be affected, as it would be for anyone confronted by this kind of comment or reaction. The need for attachment and acceptance is as real for people with memory problems as it is for anyone else.

The compounding impact of this problem is the sensitivity of those who are trying to deal with the problem. It may become very difficult to inform a person of previous total autonomy that they must wash and dress at certain times and in a certain way.

Self-care skills

His personal care started to deteriorate.

I do everything for her, toilet, shower, feed, meds everything. She lost interest and initiative.

The carer has to deal with the dilemma of ensuring that the person maintains the standards of personal care that they believe that the individual would want whilst trying to overcome the lack of awareness and consequent conflict in telling them how to do so.

Dressing can take a very long time due to the loss of skills in small tasks like closing buttons. Many people find this to be one of the most time-consuming activities of a day, and can become very tempted to take over the activity to ensure that it is done quickly and properly.

Can't put on tops and fasten buttons on my cardigans. Choose my clothes myself. Does know when to wash and dress. (*sufferer and carer*)

Can't dress himself. I choose clothes and help him dress.

I put out her clothes and she dresses.

I had to leave clothes out for him and hope he put them on. Often he put on the wrong things. We laughed about it and that relieved the frustration a lot of the time.

I put his clothes out for him and he can put them on himself.

I dress her and she mostly lets me. If she's tired she grumbles, but we usually get on with it.

Hygiene

I do everything for her, wash her and cut up food.

Legs are bad and can't get in and out of bath. Social services offered a stool, can't lower him. Got sticky things on floor of bath and two rails on side.

If in bath will wash but forgets to rinse.

I go into the shower room and remind her to shower and stuff, but she does it herself.

I had to wash him, because he was spending too much time doing it, which was his character anyway. He got really frustrated at not washing himself properly.

I have to tell him to shave, wash, shower etc.

There is an inherent danger in this area of carers taking over the skills and thus creating a potential for dependence of the sufferer on them which is not absolutely necessary. The previously discussed topic of maintaining independence in many areas also applies here. It is important to remember that each task should be considered at the time and assessed for the sufferer's ability to complete it at any level of involvement possible. For example, the sufferer may be able to wash themselves in a shower one morning, completing the whole task including rinsing and drying. The next day they may be less able and need a lot more prompting on each part of the activity to get through it. This is where it becomes very tempting for the carer to take over the task more and more, thus discouraging the sufferer from maintaining that skill. It saves time, and when there is an appointment to get to or a breakfast waiting to be eaten or generally a feeling of frustration at the slow nature of progress, it is understandable that carers wish to hurry the job along. However, this approach can lead to a quicker deterioration of ability and therefore dependence occurring before it needs to, if at all. The sufferer loses the skill very quickly if not encouraged and practised and therefore needs the carer to do the whole task for them before long. The sufferer has 'learned helplessness' (Seligman, 1992) and is potentially deteriorating before they need to.

It is impossible to make the assumption that creating dependence is the reason for a person's deterioration, as we can't tell what would have happened to the skill without the carer taking over. Therefore it is a statement made with caution that dependence can be imposed, but we can be sure that the emotional effect of loss of skill is definite. The response of many carers and sufferers to each other is defined by many theories of care when considering the reason for conflict, e.g. Malignant Social Psychology (Kitwood, 1997). This theory suggests that the activity of the carer is often influential in how people with memory problems and dementia respond in their environment. 'Disempowerment' (Kitwood, 1997, p. 46) is one aspect of this theory which is prominent in personal care. The carer can prevent the person from carrying out tasks that they can do by simply taking over, even when they have made an attempt themselves. Kitwood believed that these kinds of depersonalising behaviour on the part of professional and non-professional carers are seen as part of the caring process and are not meant as destructive or malicious, but simply as necessary to ensure safety and hygiene. Despite this he argues that this kind of approach to care promotes the loss of self-identity for the sufferer and can in fact cause them to deteriorate emotionally and practically.

This problem can be compared to the Social Model of Disability (Sayce, 2000) in that it presupposes that cultures influence our approach to care and that these cultural practices have a severe effect on an individual's situation. The model argues that disability is a socially created problem and that society makes people disabled by not adapting to individual needs, rather serving the needs of the socially acceptable normal people. For example, a person who cannot walk and needs a wheelchair is not disabled by the lack of ability to walk but by the fact that when they go out they cannot get into places because there are no ramps or lifts; and people stare at them, making them feel self-conscious and lacking in confidence to go out and feeling like they are generally just a nuisance to society. The parallels with dementia can be seen in society's need to ensure that everyone is clean, tidy and safe, even if that is at the expense of their independence and consequent loss self-esteem, skill and confidence.

How we help ourselves and each other

■ **Assess ability as normal part of routine**: Each time a personal care activity takes place, we should base assumptions of ability on the last experience as well changing quickly to react to any deterioration or improvement in the sufferer's skill at that moment.

Always assume that each task will be carried out in the uniqueness of its particular time. The outcome of the task to get washed may be the same as yesterday, but the environment, mood and thought processes may have changed for the sufferer. Recognition of these changes on a daily basis will help carers and sufferers to anticipate the need to adapt and to reduce frustration during the task.

■ **Change and adapt the task to the person's ability**: When the individual tries to use a face cloth and put soap on it and then rinse, as they did yesterday, and they cannot do any or all of these activities today, then it may be useful to break the job down from a whole task into its parts:

– Prompt to pick up the cloth – if they can't, then put it in their hand, talking and telling them what it is, and what it is for. Encourage the person to engage with the cloth as a tool for washing themselves. If they just cannot do it, then this may be the point today when you have to do this part of the task for them.

– Prompt to put soap on the cloth – if they can't, then point to the soap and explain in clear short sentences what to do with it. If they need to be instructed to put the soapy cloth to their face, then do so. If there is a lack of understanding or they just can't do it then this might be a point of assistance today.

– Prompt to rinse cloth and face and then dry in much the same way, until either the job is done or not. The carer may have had to carry it out for them. Always talk to them through each stage and inform them of the next thing to come.

This is today and tomorrow may vary; the point of this approach is about maintaining dignity, independence and a general sense of achievement rather than frustration for both sufferer and carer.

■ **Prioritise need**: It will ultimately help any stressful situation to prioritise whether or not a task itself and its process are important enough to cause friction between the sufferer and carer.

In the example of washing it could be that the withdrawal of using a cloth helps to make the activity less complicated and therefore more achievable by the sufferer. In the same example, if the sufferer objects and becomes distressed by the whole activity then the carer could consider whether it is necessary to wash at that particular time or place. This ability to compromise is the key factor in reducing the negative stimulus sometimes responsible for distress and hostility. However, it is also of concern if the sufferer continues to refuse to wash or be washed, leading to health risks like infection. In this case the carer may find that adapting the environment or approach can help to encourage the person to allow the task to take place. For example, telling the sufferer to do something may cause them to feel frustrated and then refuse. A more cajoling and encouraging attitude in the carer's request, tone of voice, and facial and body expression can be more persuasive and less humiliating to the sufferer. The room that is being used may have changed or simply become distressing to the sufferer; therefore a change of environment can help to stimulate a change in behaviour. Ironically, changes in these ways can also be the source of the distress: a move to an unfamiliar environment or an unfamiliar carer can cause a feeling of insecurity and have an impact on behaviour. The point is to remember that usually there is a reason for erratic, disturbed or changed behaviour, and in order that the sufferer and carer continue to work together calmly and respectfully it is essential to identify and resolve the source if possible.

Many aspects of daily activity are affected by dementia and its symptoms and the respondents highlight some of the experiences they have found with these.

Sleep

Neither of us ever sleeps very well and that is how it is now.

She sleeps all night.

Mum's sleep is very poor. She is up all night and then we can't keep her awake during the day.

Some nights he is up all night and others he sleeps all night.

If she sleeps all night it's OK, but I am usually awake a lot listening for her.

Her sleeping is really bad now. She is up most of the night. Then she sleeps all day despite trying to keep her awake.

Night time can become an area of contention in any care environment, as it is necessary for people to have sleep, but this is disturbed by the changing patterns of the person with dementia. It is common for people to suffer from what is often termed diurnal variation where the day is turned around – people often sleep all day instead of night. Other problems include sundowning, when the person becomes restless in the evening or at night, rather than settling down to go to bed.

The lack of sleep imposed on both carers and sufferers is apparent in the comments, and the effects are obvious as everyone knows how hard it is to remain calm and supportive when tired and stressed.

How we can help ourselves and each other

■ **Use support from statutory services**: Professional carers can help with difficult times of the day, by visiting and allowing the carer time away and the sufferer a new means of stimulation.

Respite care can also offer a time for rest and allow the sufferer and carer to have some space from the strains of a stressful lack of sleep. However, respite care can sometimes upset routines, so its usefulness varies for individuals.

Use medical advice about the use of medication at strategic times if the problems are extreme. It is not acceptable ethically to administer sedating medication simply to make things easier for the carer, but it is understandable and acceptable to use medication for the psychological and behavioural control of symptoms. This in turn can help the sufferer to feel better emotionally and functionally, therefore reducing distress.

■ **Establish a routine as far as possible**: Time for sleeping during the day can be restricted by a stimulating activity schedule like going out or attending a day centre.

Adapting the day has been the key theme throughout this book and it does not change here. However, what does change is the approach to adaptation. The need for sleep is essential for all living creatures and therefore it is a priority that people with dementia and carers get enough rest and sleep. The routine of sleep at night and awake with cat naps during the day can be established as the adaptation itself. The approach to calming the environment in the evening and stimulating during the day can help to ensure that a pattern is effective.

Using the toilet

Using the toilet is also an area of social embarrassment and can lead to people coming into conflict with each other. The basic need to go to the toilet and awareness of the need can be affected by physical problems, like physical disability or lack of control caused by infection. Therefore it is important to ensure that incontinence is not assumed to be normal under any circumstances. When a person becomes incontinent, its cause should always be investigated, as there will always be a reason. It may be that the reason is untreatable or irresolvable, like physical disability, but infections and routines of going to the toilet can always be resolved. It may be that the person is only incontinent because of not being prompted to go the toilet (or taken if necessary) on a regular basis. The institution of a pattern can often reverse a potentially distressing and time-consuming task in the symptoms of dementia and associated care. The introduction of antibiotics because of diagnosed infection can also provide a remedy to a painful problem which can contribute to other behavioural disturbances.

The carers discuss this issue below. No one finds it an easy aspect of care, and it is one which they identify to be a critical aspect of their ability to cope.

> She tells me when she needs to go to the toilet.

> Sometimes she doesn't get to the toilet on time. Seen by the nurse, we had to record when and measure the water, she didn't like that. Now she wears incontinence pants. It's usually if she can't get to a toilet, like when shopping.

The sufferer expresses her feeling as best she can, demonstrating another reason to prevent incontinence if possible.

> I don't like that [incontinence] (*sufferer*)

> Sometimes she struggles to use the toilet properly, needs to be guided.

> He got to the stage where he didn't know what the toilet was for. He had bowel problems and then it became really difficult because he began to get irritated by me taking him there. We were very often in a mess. The nurse tried to help with meds but it didn't help other than make him incontinent more.

It is important to remember that incontinence is not inevitable and can at least be delayed, if not prevented, by assuming that any onset should be investigated and if possible treated.

> He is not incontinent.

However, when it does become a problem it causes enormous distress and concern, and both sufferer and carer need support to cope with the effects.

> She won't sit on the toilet and she's doubly incontinent and this goes all over the floor. I can't get her to sit down. She used to put faeces down the radiators and stuff. She takes inco pads off. I found big inco pants and she keeps them on better. She slipped onto the floor on the Kylie sheets, so I buy these nappy-type bed covers. Sometimes she's nasty, and will not put them on. So I spend the night checking on her.

> If he got incontinent I think he would have to go into a home. I would feel a failure if he had to.

How we can help ourselves and each other

■ **Understand the embarrassment caused by toileting issues**: It is humiliating for anyone to be taken to the toilet and told to sit down, and then to use the toilet in front of another person. Even worse is when the person with memory problems is taken, undressed and sat on the toilet. It is easy for carers to become complacent about this feeling, as expressed by respondents above, and to assume that they need to take over this activity to ensure it is carried out properly.

It may well be necessary to do so, but the humiliation felt by all can be alleviated by two main points:

– Never assume that the person can't do it themselves; always use prompting methods described above for personal care.
– Try to be as discreet as possible and explain all activity before it happens. For example, simple instruction and guidance on the fact that the toilet is here and that clothes need to be removed, etc.

■ **Establish an individualised pattern for toileting**: The bladder and bowels can establish a pattern if trained, and it is possible to maintain someone's continence by simply finding the individual's pattern. Constipation and diarrhoea can cause pain and can be present as a result of certain medications, dehydration, poor dietary balance or general physical illness. It is important to monitor and record intake and output to ensure an accurate record of any patterns or disturbances in patterns of eliminating.

This will involve monitoring and recording when the sufferer uses the toilet and whether there are any stimulants which promote or hinder a regular routine. For example, if having bran in porridge causes loose stools, then perhaps fibre has to be gained from a different source. If having to wait to be taken to the toilet for too long causes incontinence then the person has to be taken earlier.

Once a pattern is identified then it may be possible to change it if necessary, but ultimately the need is to work around it, ensuring that the support needed to get to the toilet at appropriate times is accommodated.

■ **Assume incontinence is not normal**: If a person is incontinent it may be due to muscular problems, previous surgery or simply infection. The point is that it is not an automatic problem for people with dementia or memory problems, and should always be investigated.

Access to support in assessing this can be found in statutory services via the GP and health or social care professionals. Full assessment of the person's ability to maintain continence will be carried out by a continence specialist and action taken to support the carer in doing so, or in some cases coping with the effects of incontinence.

The use of incontinence pads can have inherent risks of infection and is generally undesirable – often the reason given by the respondents as a reason for not being able to continue to cope.

It is possible to develop a hygienic and respectful approach to managing continence, involving the use of regular changes, cleansing thoroughly and drying the skin afterwards. With the use of a respectful approach and an adaptable routine as already advised, it can be a problem dealt with more effectively than the carers may give themselves credit for.

Eating and drinking

Eating and drinking are a particular problem if the person with memory problems or dementia lives alone. They are not monitored and it is very easy to deteriorate physically very quickly due to a lack of nutrition without it being noticed. Professional and non-professional carers need to develop an acute awareness of this aspect of care for those living alone so that potentially life-threatening problems are prevented.

Otherwise, eating and drinking patterns do change often, but can be managed by carers adapting to the person's individual needs.

She wasn't eating and lost loads of weight.

I do everything for her: wash her and cut up food.

Can't make tea or cook. Eats less but usually eats everything, knife and fork becoming a problem.

We feed and change him as he is doubly incontinent. He walks about a lot and won't sit down to eat. Eats well and usually takes meds. We give him a lot of space to walk around. He hits things and then calms down. The carer sleeps in the room with him and we usually have the same carers.

She eats and drinks fine.

I've always liked my food. Tastes haven't changed (*sufferer*)

I had to keep encouraging him to sit at the table, but he ate himself when he was sat down.

He eats and drinks too much. He's had a meal then an hour later he is in the kitchen getting himself more food. He's put on a stone and a half in weight over the last six months. He does what I tell him.

She still eats but doesn't recognise the cutlery and needs help.

How we can help ourselves and each other

■ **Monitor those living alone**: On regular visits weigh the person and encourage clothes changing whilst there to be able to assess the weight. It is possible to use some scales of measurement, such as the Body Mass Index, to indicate the appropriateness of their weight. However, it is much better to measure the current weight patterns of the individual against those of the past. If a person has always been underweight then the problem may be associated with the dementia only if they begin to lose even more. Other factors which suggest excessive weight loss and dehydration are unusual skin dryness or tearing, loss of energy, loss of appetite and recurring infection or constipation, etc. – essentially, anything out of the ordinary for the individual should be monitored closely and assessed for its effect overall.

It may be useful to encourage social eating at a day centre or to arrange meals on wheels to try to ensure that food is eaten regularly.

Shopping trips together with sufferer and carer may help to decide which foods the person is more likely to eat and therefore can be left in their home to access easily.

■ **Adapt eating and drinking patterns**: The use of routines can help to ensure that the person is eating a regular healthy diet, but it is possible that full meals at particular times of day are no longer tolerated.

It is possible to ensure adequate nutrition by adapting the food or the presentation of it.

Have snacks available when needed to reduce the potential for getting hungry and insisting on unhealthy food. The use of little sandwich trays or fruit or crackers with cheese already made up is an examples of nutritious and enjoyable food being available. This can be extended to whole meals being cooked and kept in the fridge for picking at, or eating when ready.

Use of crockery and cutlery which assists the person to eat independently will affect their acceptance of the need to eat. If it seems impossible to pick up food with a fork then a person is less likely to do it. Adaptable tools can be accessed through statutory services and in specialist shops for care. Voluntary organisations, discussed in other chapters, will be able to direct carers to local outlets who sell these implements.

If there are problems with eating too much then the availability of certain foods in the house may need to be restricted. Buying one chocolate bar and leaving chunks out at a time where they can be accessed will be a healthier approach than leaving out all the chocolate bars, as well as less confrontational than trying to persuade the person not to eat them all at once.

The following advice concerns general tips for a good diet. There are obvious issues with undertaking this kind of diet for carers and people with memory problems, but they offer a basis from which to work. There are also differences between the nutritional needs of individuals influenced by age, sex, size or illness.

Some more specific information on some common dietary problems for sufferers and carers is relevant to a loss of appetite, swallowing difficulties, changes in taste or lack of comprehension or sensory stimulation. Some key tips may help: see the box below.

Eight tips on healthy eating (Food Standards Agency, 2005)

- Base your meals on starchy foods: rice, pasta, potatoes; wholegrain versions if possible
- Eat loads of fruit and vegetables
- Eat more fish, especially oily fish like mackerel, sardines or salmon
- Eat less saturated fat – meat pies, sausages, pastry, butter, hard cheese, coconut oil

This is *a lot* of fat:
20 g fat or more per 100 g
5 g saturates or more per 100 g

This is *a little* fat:
3 g fat or less per 100 g
1 g saturates or less per 100 g
10 g sugars or more per 100 g is *a lot* of sugar
2 g sugars or less per 100 g is *a little* sugar

- Try to eat less salt – no more than 6 grams a day – often described as sodium on packets

This is *a lot* of salt:
1.25 g salt or more per 100 g
0.5 g sodium or more per 100 g

This is *a little* salt:
0.25 g salt or less per 100 g
0.1 g sodium or less per 100 g

- Get active and try to be a healthy weight
- Drink more water (6–8 glasses of water a day). Reduce or limit alcohol. Women can drink up to 2–3 units of alcohol a day and men up to 3–4 units a day without significant risk to their health.
- Don't skip breakfast

Some more tips:

■ Try to add as much nutrition to small snacks as regularly as possible. Use milk in drinks and prepare food in an attractive way.
■ Avoid using the same ingredients and dishes all the time, as people will become bored. Introduce new but mild tasting items to snacks.
■ Buy and use soft foods like mashed potatoes, pastas with sauce, fish in tins, rice pudding, custard, powdered milky drinks, jam, honey etc.
■ Only liquidise food if necessary. If someone has problems with swallowing then they may be at risk of choking – ensure they are urgently checked over by a doctor or dietitian.
■ To accommodate tastes and taste changes ensure a supply of varied ingredients and be prepared to alter the menu. Offer different and stimulating tastes as alternatives. Keep the mouth clean.

Medication with food issues

Medication compliance is an area which can be influenced by a person's reluctance to take any food or drink. The carer must consider issues of consent and capacity when giving medication in food, as this practice is neither ethical nor legal. There are exceptions to this rule, and in some cases professionals can administer medication disguised as food or in drinks, but only under strict criteria and guidelines and only if it is shown to be in the best interests of the sufferer.

The main ethical reasons for this are that people should have choice as far as possible and this includes those with memory problems. The Capacity to Consent Act 2005 has gone some way to promoting this by ensuring that everyone, regardless of diagnosis has the right to choose and to be assumed competent, until proven otherwise. Practical reasons for not giving prescribed medication in food and drink include the problem that the food may not be eaten fully, and therefore it is difficult to know how much the person took. Also the person may refuse the food as it tastes bad, and this then impacts on eating habits. Lastly, the chemical structure of the medication can be changed by the food, making it either dangerous or ineffective.

Monitor skin condition

It is very important to monitor people's skin condition when they are in a position of poor mobility, lack awareness about their own health, are not eating and drinking well, have certain medications, suffer from diabetes or decreased circulation, or are incontinent. People who have dementia or memory problems can have some, all or none of these issues, but as a carer it is vital to be alert to the potential problems associated with them.

Skin is very vulnerable and can become sore and break down under these conditions into ulcers or pressure sores. Consequently, an individual who fits any or some of these descriptions should be closely watched and then treated in the following way:

- Check vulnerable pressure points daily: buttocks, back, shoulders, elbows, knees, heels, under breasts, faces or heads, groin area, or any area of the body which is constantly under this kind of pressure. Look for discolouration, any signs of pain like grimacing, or loss of feeling on touch.
- If discolouration is found then action should be taken immediately to prevent skin breakdown. Professional consultation at this point may involve assessment using a Waterlow (2005) score to identify risk.
- Immediate or preventative action involves gentle cleansing of the area with water and non-irritant cleaning solutions, e.g. anti-allergy or non-perfumed products.
- Dry well without rubbing.
- Apply barrier cream, unless skin is already broken (in this case a professional treatment or dressing needs to be prescribed).
- Do not apply talc or irritant creams.
- Consult an expert in tissue viability immediately or a professional involved in care.

Assume the need to be attentive for expression of pain

Remember that for anyone pain is very different and can be felt in different ways as well as with varying tolerance. For a person with memory problems or dementia this lack of clarity can be compounded by being unable to express the existence, nature or severity of any pain.

It is important to acknowledge and investigate any verbal attempts to identify pain. For example, any communication being used in a stressed sounding way during a walk down stairs could be the person trying to identify limb pain.

Pain from infection, constipation and diarrhoea can all be alleviated by the carer's awareness of its existence and consequent actions.

McClean (2000) discusses pain and management of it with people who have dementia and identifies key areas for carers to be aware of: what is pain, how does the person identify it and how do we manage it? He offers an insight into more professional concerns, but the following points are key to the general awareness of pain issues.

Non-verbal expressions of pain can be seen by keen observation of changes in reaction of the face, body language or tone of voice: for example, lying with legs curled up, spitting out food when being fed or hitting out at the carer when being moved. It is possible that pain is causing an indirect reaction and should always be investigated.

Chronic or long-lasting pain can be less easy to identify due to the behaviours not changing suddenly. Some indicators of general and constant pain are depression, anger, poor sleep patterns, impaired ability to mobilise and drug dependency.

Generally it will be possible to monitor a person with memory problems for pain in day-to-day activities, and the use of daily recording behaviours and reactions will help to identify them more effectively.

If pain is detected as a reason for a particular behaviour, professional assessment from a pain specialist is essential. Many medications and treatments may be possible to help, but there are safety issues and risks to be considered when giving a person with dementia or memory problems any medication.

Social life

A social life can seem like it is a thing of the past when a family or person is suffering from dementia. The loss of social skills, awareness, interests and functioning, as well as sometimes disruptive behaviour, can inhibit the person and carers from trying to continue with their social pattern. However, it can be seen here that some aspects of socialisation can remain intact and new ones can be created or adapted.

> She stopped reading and embroidery. Picks up newspaper and puts it down again; TV is on but she doesn't really watch it. We go to the pub every weekend, I go to my allotment, she goes to day centre once a week and her friends once a week. We go on bus trips and we go down town.

> Don't do what we used to, but still go out and go on coach trips.

> Used to go out a lot for meals, but only occasionally now. I have to think ahead. We go with some friends that are in the same position and we go out for walks and stuff. We don't go out like we did and we don't do our camping any more. We go on coach tours now and that's OK and we go with our friends.

We haven't really changed. We go down the club on a Saturday night. We go on day trips with Alzheimer's Society and their support group. We go for the shopping and stuff. She can't go on her own.

I go to a day centre and I like that, I can have a chat and stuff. They've got time for you. Don't want to go more than once a week (*sufferer*)

He used to enjoy going to MIND and had a sitting service which he enjoyed, but then he became hostile with them and MIND had to stop. We still managed to go out and to friends, but I knew when to stop.

We only go shopping now. We used to go out all the time and he was out most nights. He wouldn't cope with any of these things any more. He enjoys the day centre, says he wishes I could come. I try to keep busy by going to the gym and seeing friends. I get emotional support from my daughter. I am spiritual but don't go to church. It helps and I don't see this as a burden but a learning curve. I have applied for a part-time post to give me something interesting to do. We can't go on holiday any more because he wanders off.

Mum goes to day centre four days now. She is always happy to go and comes back fine. I go out when she is at the day centre. We take her everywhere and that is difficult but you have to learn how to deal with her. She won't eat in a restaurant, but I just have to accept that and not worry. In toilets we are in for ages and I have to keep shouting out to people we won't be long.

The sufferer and carer can benefit greatly from socialising if it is adapted to their ability, thus preventing them from being under-stimulated and potentially depressed.

How we can help ourselves and each other

■ **Maintain social contacts**: The need for social contact is essential for most human beings and it helps to enhance a sense of belongingness. However, when affected by memory loss or dementia, people and their carers are often faced with rejection through poor understanding and lack of accommodation in public places of perceived difficult behaviour.

Despite this many of the people interviewed in this study were able to identify the adaptations they made to ensure that social contact of some kind was maintained.

■ **General principles involve**:
  – Always try to understand that onlookers don't understand the problems and may need reassurance and explanation. Alternatively, they may just

reject any involvement and this can be very distressing for the sufferer and carer and just another example of loss.

– Dealing with loss is very difficult, and any carer, professional or non-professional should seek support in doing so from health and social care professionals or voluntary organisational support.

– Adapt where you go and when. For example, try to avoid busy town centres on a Saturday afternoon and instead try to walk around shops or parks or go on day trips on calm days when they are not busy. Visit friends and relatives who do understand and will be able to accommodate the changing behaviours without causing worry and distress.

– Use specialist support offered by carers groups, day centres etc. to get peer support and understanding.

References

Archibald, C. (2003) *People with Dementia in Acute Hospitals. A Practical Guide for Clinical Support Workers.* Dementia Services Development centre, University of Stirling.

Food Standards Agency (2005) *8 Tips for Eating Well.* http://www.eatwell. gov.uk/healthydiet/8tips/.

Grealy, J., McMullen, H. and Grealy, J. (2005) *Dementia Care: a Practical Photographic Guide.* Blackwell Publishing, Oxford.

Kitwood, T. (1997) *Dementia Reconsidered: the Person Comes First.* Open University Press, Maidenhead.

McClean W (2000) Practice guide for pain management for people with dementia. Conference on Pain Management, Centre for Research on Families and Relationships. http://www.crfr.ac.uk/DementiaNetwork/Recognising%20P ain%20in%20the%20Elderly.doc.

Office for National Statistics (2000) *Psychiatric Morbidity among Adults Living in Private Households, 2000.* http://www.statistics.gov.uk/downloads/ theme_health/psychmorb.pdf.

Sayce, L. (2000) *From Psychiatric Patient to Citizen: Overcoming Discrimination and Social Exclusion.* Macmillan Press, London.

Seligman, M. (1992) *Helplessness.* Freeman, New York.

Waterlow, J. (2005) *Waterlow Pressure Ulcer Prevention Manual.* http://www. judy-waterlow.co.uk/waterlow_downloads.htm.

CHAPTER 8

The effect of dementia on thinking processes

Learning points on the effect of being unable to process thoughts and memories effectively:

- The effect of changes in thinking and communication
- How we can help ourselves and each other by understanding behaviours and using alternative routines and activities
- The use of philosophical approaches to therapeutic interventions, including validation therapy, positive person work and psychosocial interventions
- Younger people with dementia, the use of Admiral Nurses and other therapeutic interventions

Communicating with disturbed thought processes

Aspects of how the effect of memory problems or dementia affects a person's ability to communicate, rationalise, make decisions, learn, adapt and generally retain information are fundamental to all issues of care and are affected by the disturbed thought processes commonly found in people with dementia. The other chapters are all associated with this process in some way, as the problems and changes in an individual's behaviour can ultimately be associated with their thought processes, or cognition.

Consideration of the definitions of dementia reminds people that the main area of concern is the loss of intellectual capacity. This does not simply mean the loss of the ability to do maths equations or crossword puzzles; it includes a functional deterioration of all activities of the brain, including memory, learning, language abilities, reading and writing and the ability to interpret information given. Within a diagnosis it is also important to remember the changes in behavioural, emotional, psychological and social aspects of the person, but this chapter is concerned with the effects of changes in thinking.

Many of the respondents in the interviews expressed feelings of frustration at a lack of communication, loss of ability to carry out activities or the restrictions that were imposed on their life plans. This can be explained by the inability of the sufferer and carer to express themselves to each other in many cases, but also could be influenced by the sufferers' reduced ability to retain information about tasks they have always done or new activities that they could learn.

> When she can't do things she gets frustrated.

> I thought I was prepared, but I wasn't. I had to learn to live with it.

> His mood was so nice sometimes and at others he got so frustrated because he didn't know what was going on. He got so frustrated with everyone, not like him.

> He lost responsibility for his actions.

> She wonders when her mum is coming down and where her baby is lately. She can't take a message on the phone.

> I don't always remember. I think I should be able to remember this and it gets to me. I have cried, I think I'm not very clever and it gets me down. If I have to do anything they have to tell me (*sufferer*)

> She doesn't recognise any of us, won't even answer to Mum.

> Constantly repeating the same question.

> He got to the stage where he didn't know what the toilet was for.

> She won't sit on the toilet and is doubly incontinent. I can't get her to sit down.

> She doesn't get angry.

> She is often agitated and it is not sparked by anything in particular. She paces around and gets very anxious. Some days you can't do anything with her.

> We don't communicate any more because he can't understand what I am saying to him and he doesn't tell me things. It is very frustrating.

> I feel irritated when I can't remember.

> She doesn't believe what we tell her.

> Mum gets frustrated by her own inability to do things, or not knowing what is going on.

> I get upset and frustrated when I can't see what I have to do next and I have to ask them. They are very good and help me, but I feel I ought to be doing it myself (*sufferer*)

> Sometimes I feel very frustrated because we can't do what we planned for our retirement.

I think I'm getting better, although sometimes I feel a bit yuk (*sufferer*)

Sometimes she realises what she has done and says sorry.

He gets upset to not be able to help.

As can be seen in the comments there is a lot of tension and anxiety as a result of this loss of ability to think through activities and carry them out. In many cases the frustration is associated with sheer disappointment at not being able to understand instructions, or simply because the two people find it impossible to communicate what they are trying to say.

These problems are not exclusive to the personal relationships of the sufferer, but also affect their public lives. People who are still working and driving, for example, are faced with the further embarrassment and humiliation of losing intellectual capacity in less protected places. Associated with this change is the potentially less compassionate adaptation of the sufferer's environment when faced with the employer's concern for health and safety and general production of work. The loss of another role can only cause the sufferer distress and have the compounding effect of reducing mental stimulation, which is something they may actually crave at this stage.

He got early retirement from work on sick grounds. He didn't want it but accepted that he would have a better quality of life.

She started making mistakes at work and her employers were concerned about her.

She was told not to drive but kept on because she wanted to keep her job. She couldn't do manoeuvres and was stopping at junctions too long and stuff.

He was driving too long and eventually DVLA refused to renew his license.

The reaction to these changes in functioning are incredibly powerful and can be demonstrated here in a positive way. It is possible to manage to be compassionate and yet still achieve the goal of completing an activity with someone who is aggressive or hostile. The need for carers to understand the reasons for the behaviour are key to this approach and have been part of the overall approach of the whole of this book. In this case it is especially vital to learn to adapt based on the understanding that the sufferer is reacting to something.

She started a day centre and seems to enjoy it. She told me she is doing stuff and I had to learn to go along with her, because she thought she had done these things.

I went down and they had him on the floor with five people on him. I leant down and touched him on the head and he was crying; then he was fine.

I put out her clothes and she dresses herself.

Feel better now because I can go out, although not on my own. I feel better and we do everything together (*sufferer*)

We let him wander about and calm himself down. If he is out of routine, tired, wet, there are too many people around, doesn't like the dark because of the shadows and hallucinations, in pain or just fed up then he gets aggressive.

Just now he will understand if you speak slowly.

Sometimes I know what is wrong, like when she comes back form MIND and has had to sit on the bus for ages. She is agitated.

I could tell when he was getting worked up and needed to go to the toilet or something. We were often in situations when we were both crying, not knowing what to do and I just had to get help, cause he was too upset and he didn't understand.

I can mostly tell what he is trying to say even when he became unable to talk properly.

He goes for walks most days and that keeps him calm usually.

I had to change how I talk to him, like saying someone is coming to see him rather than someone is here to fetch you.

So far it's all going to plan and he does what I ask him to do.

We have to change the pattern daily 'cause she is different everyday.

Sometimes he got frustrated, but I just distracted him.

Often we went to church, even now, and he is very settled.

We got married a year ago. He was deemed able to make a decision and we did it.

My husband can make her laugh, and she is often cheered up by an ice cream.

The main action that can be taken from these comments is that the carer reacted to what they felt the sufferer's worries and concerns actually are, rather than assuming that the behaviour is simply aggression which needs to be managed. Understanding and communication with the person are limited by the loss of the ability to understand instructions or to express feelings. This can be overcome by familiarity with the individual and a general adaptation of approach, as necessary.

The Skilled Helper Model (Gerard, 1998) offers the carer an approach to develop the relationship as a means to an end. This can empower the person with memory problems in the use of any therapeutic approach. It requires the use of three stages:

- **Stage 1**: Identify the problem with the sufferer.
- **Stage 2**: Establish goals and outcomes with the sufferer.
- **Stage 3**: Identify/plan activities of how to do it.

The three stages must involve the person with the memory problems or dementia to ensure its empowering nature. It is assumed that the more involved people are, the more likely it is that the plan will have some success.

This model is simply a structural approach to try to see the changes in thinking as something which can be accommodated and worked with. It assumes that compliance with its structure is straightforward, but (as is demonstrated by the interview respondents) nothing is ever simple in a caring relationship. Despite this, it does offer a basis from which to start which may help carers to approach the problems they face differently.

How we can help ourselves and each other

- **Approach problem behaviours as behaviours to be understood**: The changing capacity of the sufferer to undertake thinking activities is inevitable and needs to be seen as an aspect of memory problems and dementia which the individual needs help to sustain and possibly even improve. In order to achieve this it would be necessary for professional and non-professional carers to be able to assess the person's likes and dislikes, intellectual capacity and general reactions on a daily basis. This requires some skills and a lot of patience.

  It is also important to remember that the carer is not infallible and will become frustrated by repetitive questioning and behaviours and by the lack of progress so often associated with those people who have cognitive problems. However, the outlook is not all bleak. It is possible to communicate with someone who has little cognitive functioning and continue a certain level of connection.

  Killick and Allan (2001) suggest that the change in the relationship can be frightening and carers often come to the conclusion that their loved ones have just disappeared. This means of course that there is no need to be intimate or to understand, because they can remove themselves from the personal situation. The professional carer has this perspective already in their arsenal of defences. If both can see the person still living behind the loss of character, personality, ability and familiarity, then it should be possible to see the new person emerging. This may not be the individual that they want or indeed have loved, but this is still a person with feelings and thoughts and actions which require assistance and compassion.

■ **Use non-verbal communication and body language**: Learn the significance of behaviour by recording and examining patterns and their stimulus. Reactions to a stimulus, like seeing hallucinations, may be repetitive but not obvious. A person in pain may be aggressive when being assisted to get out of bed due to arthritis or simply having a cramp in the leg. If a person is crying it is quite inevitable that they are distressed by something. Spend time tracing back their actions/activities/stimulus to see if there is something new or unusual happening.

■ **Learn about the individual, their likes and dislikes**: This biographical approach is recognised as particularly useful when people have behavioural traits. For example, a man who has worked on night shifts in a dark coal mine may be very prone to waking during the night and trying to do his work. The lack of understanding of this motivation can lead to extreme frustration for the carer and an inability to resolve the issue. An approach which may help is to accommodate the working pattern as far as possible and try to gradually reduce the so-called working hours each night. Leave the light on in the room if the darkness is stimulating the night memory.

This approach can also, however, be misleading as it assumes that people's preferences do not change throughout life. For example, because a person with memory problems liked Tom Jones's music in the past, that does not mean that they will like it now. In order to use a biographical approach the carer must be cautious to remember that opinions change and tastes change. The other problem with this approach is that there may be no obvious way to gain an accurate history if the person with memory problems is not able to recall and there are no close relatives or friends to ask.

■ **Adapt reactions, environment and stimulus**: Many behaviours and reactions are either influenced or affected by the person's environment or the stimulation they are exposed to. The awareness of the room that a person is in can often give clues to the reasons why they are doing whatever they are doing at that time. Many care facilities are becoming more attuned to this and have used colour psychology, room layout and familiar items in an effort to make the person's environment more comfortable and relaxing for them as an individual.

If the sufferer reacts consistently in a defensive, aggressive, hostile or withdrawn way without any obvious reason, then it is very possible that some kind of stimulus has initiated this change in behaviour. The activity of trying to stimulate someone by playing a game may be too overwhelming and cause the individual to react. It is easy, when the carer understands this reaction, to be able to adapt the game. For example don't play chess, but play card games etc., depending on the individual's ability.

Daily activity can include one-to-one discussions for short periods, multi-sensory environments to increase alertness or relaxation, active listening to improve communication rather than ignoring or disregarding what seems like non-communication from the sufferer, adaptable routines and general empathic approaches to talking.

■ **Use therapeutic and social activities to stimulate, prevent distress and to distract**: There are many therapeutic approaches which can be applied when caring for someone with a memory problem and these are not exclusive to therapists. It is possible to use aspects of an approach in the day-to-day activities of any carer. However, it would be a mistake to assume that the use of the philosophy of these theories makes the carer a therapist. They are very complex and in their therapeutic use require great skill to use appropriately and ethically.

However, the philosophy and principles of each can be used to enhance the relationship and can be examined in more detail by use of the references offered here. Examples include:

– *Validation therapy* (Feil, 1993): This therapy was devised as one of the first practical uses of person-centred theory. It acknowledges the person with dementia and their feelings as significant rather than gobbledegook. The emphasis is on the carer to ensure that the person's needs are identified and facilitated. It is claimed that this approach will alleviate distress and consequent behaviours. The main approach is always to regard an action, expression or behaviour as something to be understood and to assist the person in expressing it and resolving it.

– *Resolution therapy* (Stokes, 2000): This approach is about seeing challenging behaviours as needs to be met, not problems to be managed. The humanistic understanding of people with dementia in this case is that they have plenty to say which is often dismissed when they say it. The impaired communication is often misinterpreted and therefore seen as behaviour to be dealt with and managed rather than understood and prevented. This therapy argues that understanding what disturbed or challenging behaviour means to a person is the key to reducing the associated distress. Day-to-day use of resolution therapy may be to constantly re-frame or re-examine the behaviour in different contexts and try to see it is a different way. For example, if a person will not sit on the toilet to use it, it may be that on further investigation their inability to see the toilet and make the connection with sitting has led to a fear of falling. A possible solution, then, could be to the person orientate by showing them the toilet and consistently, clearly and simply offering reassurance and guidance on the process of sitting down.

– *Positive person work*: This has its origins in a humanistic background and personhood specifically identified by Kitwood and Bredin (1992). Positive person work (PPW) is about seeing dementia as an accumulation of issues, and the following equation is its origin.

$$\text{Dementia} = \text{Personality} + \text{Biography} + \text{Neurological impairment} + \text{Social psychology} + \text{Physical health}$$

The effect and influence of all these components of a person's life are the reason people behave in the way they do. The authors argue that it is not as simple as having a disease called dementia. Kitwood and many authors since have argued that dementia is not just illness and pathology, and knowing this is the key to helping people to live with it. It is suggested that problem behaviours are only problems because of poor interpretation, and therefore intervention, by the carer. Understanding the meaning behind the behaviour will lead to enhanced relationship development.

Malignant social psychology is a non-malicious but intrinsic part of the experience of dementia for many sufferers because it includes well-meaning care which strips them of their individuality, e.g. telling people off, shouting, humiliating and creating dependence. The use of PPW requires that carers are aware that this behaviour can be destructive. The aim of the equation and its theory is to move away from an attitude which means using any depersonalising care strategy at the expense of the person's self-esteem or respect, or personhood, so that the job is completed. PPW includes changing carer behaviours and environments from malignant social psychology to recognition, negotiation, collaboration, facilitating etc.

The day-to-day approach to care can be influenced by this approach and it is simply about accepting the need to see each individual and their actions as part of their complex coping skills. For example, if an individual becomes distressed by being given some food, then it is possible that they don't like the food, or they don't feel physically able to eat it, or they are not hungry, or they are in pain, or they are uncomfortable in that environment etc. There are many potential explanations for a reaction. The point of a person-centred approach is that the distress displayed is real and there is a reason. The need to identify that reason is the most important thing, and then the distress can be resolved.

Psychosocial interventions

The use of the stress vulnerability model for psychoses (Zubin and Spring, 1977) may be an area for potential development of therapeutic approaches in dementia care. This is far from a resolved issue and little research has been completed regarding its transferability to dementia sufferers' needs and the adaptations that would inevitably be required. However, it is important to remember that people with dementia also suffer from psychoses, and they also have the same vulnerabilities in their emotional and family lives as those without dementia. It is also important to note the mistakes of the emergence of this theory, in that it imposed an enormous burden of guilt and feelings of blame for the onset of illness on the families concerned. This is not how it should be used for people with dementia, but it should simply researched as a means of assisting social groups and families to learn how to help each other based on their day-to-day lives.

Therefore it is justified to discuss the potential benefits of this and to promote their research and development as basic principles which could be used for the benefit of people with memory problems or dementia. The model applied to dementia could suggest that the intrinsic vulnerability is caused by dementia. The experienced problem emotions and behaviours are related to coping skills, strategies, resources and perceived stress. If this is found to be true, then interventions can include identifying the issues and developing effective, realistic coping skills. These offer a range of interventions which address the needs of the person with dementia and the carer by using strategies of reducing the effect of the stress of the illness and thus having a positive effect on the quality of care provided. Marriot *et al.* (2000), cited in Keady *et al.* (2003), demonstrate a reduction in distress, depression and disturbed behaviour by use of expressed emotion (EE) and family therapy work. EE is a measure of verbal report and tone of voice. A high EE score suggests a high level of emotional over-involvement, hostility and criticism. Many studies, including that of Kavanagh (1992), cited in Thomson and Mathias (2000), shows a relationship between high EE and high levels of strain and distress and the relapse of symptoms. Any indication of high EE suggests a need to develop a new and more appropriate emotional response.

Cognitive Behavioural Therapy concentrates on what is referred to as errors of thinking and consequent actions. It is mainly used for people with anxiety, which Wands *et al.* (1990) claim is present in 38% of people with dementia. It is also used for people with depression, which Reifler (1986) and Wagner (1997) (both cited in Keady *et al.*, 2003) claim is present in 30% of people with dementia. People with dementia have a multi-faceted illness or problems and CBT may be able to help to identify the thoughts behind their behaviours or to identify behaviours and new coping strategies for them. If shown to be appropriate, this kind of work, as adapted, could bring benefits of maintaining independence longer, alleviating distress and depression, increasing socialisation and developing relationships in difficult situations. However, if used inappropriately it could be negatively affected by long-term intervention and dependence, non-acceptance of issues, inability to retain information and the loss of reality, because some negative thoughts are actually realistic. For example, dementia is devastating and cannot be problem-solved away.

Younger people with dementia

People who are younger when affected by memory problems or dementia will have specific needs which are different from those in older age groups. This book has not identified particular age groups so far because the underlying philosophy is about the individual and not societal groups. However, it is important to mention the intricacies of problems particularly related to this group of sufferers.

Different roles in people's younger years include spouses, children, work and general social activities which younger, fitter people participate in. The onset of memory problems or dementia at this stage of life can have huge financial implications for a family, or emotional disturbances for children or relationship breakdowns. There is a need to recognise the severity of these problems in relation to the individuals involved, which could be addressed through therapies used for non-dementia sufferers, such as counselling (including conflict resolution in family therapy) or skills training to prevent loss of skill in an activity or job.

Admiral Nurses

These nurses are professionally trained, based on a model of care which was initiated in the mid-1980s by the carer family of a man called Joseph Levy, who was a yachtsman in his working life – hence the name 'Admiral'. These professionals provide a support service for carers through consultancy or casework. The theory of their work is based on the assumption that supporting the carer means consequent quality care for the person with dementia. In reality, not many statutory services have Admiral Nurses in their employment, but a move towards more focused professional posts, which could be along these lines or that of a dementia specialist, suggests that it might be a potential role development for the future.

Whilst all of these approaches to therapy for people with memory problems and dementia are potentially useful, it is possible to use the philosophical background from which they came whilst still trying to live with dementia during any development and research. Exploring problems by using a person-centred approach and considering the sufferer's emotions as a priority is an appropriate means of trying to set goals and help people deal with the emotions and behaviours of, and reactions to, dementia.

Other therapies include reminiscence and reality orientation, music, art, doll therapy and life story work. This is simply an overview of the potential for therapeutic work with people who have memory problems or dementia and it is possible for professional and non-professional carers to take part in training in these roles through voluntary organisations and educational institutions.

The benefits of these approaches are obvious in that they have the potential to provide the sufferer and carer with a means of expression, and they do not dwell on problems but instead stimulate positive aspects of life and therefore assist people to live a resourceful life, despite the disability or illness effects imposed upon them. However, it is also important to remember that these techniques do not exclude accepting that the emotional turmoil and devastation caused by the symptoms of dementia are very real and require more in-depth treatment and support. The loss of focus on the medical role in the use of medication is to be avoided. The medical approach offers people relief from extreme anguish and is an area where research into cause and treatment is intense.

Another inherent danger in trying to live with dementia in this way lies in the carer being inexperienced or unwilling to accept advice and support. Missing information in techniques of care and an inability to see the side effects can lead to an even more distressing experience for all involved. The effect of assuming expertise in these approaches is that the relationship can be so badly affected that it causes withdrawal and intensifying of the problems.

It is therefore essential that all carers, professional and non-professional, gain some kind of support, training and guidance in any approach they plan to use. Even if the use is limited and basic it may be that a simple reflective chat with someone who has used it more often will enlighten the carer in its use.

References

Feil, N. (1993) *The Validation Breakthrough: Simple Techniques for Communicating with People with Alzheimer's-Type Dementia*. Health Professionals Press, London.

Gerard, E. (1998) *The Skilled Helper: a Problem Management Approach to Helping*, 6th edn. Brooks Cole Publishing, California.

Keady, J., Clarke, C. L. and Adams, T. (2003) *Community Mental Health Nursing and Dementia Care – Practice Perspectives*. Open University Press, Maidenhead.

Killick, J. and Allan, K. (2001) *Communication and the Care of People with Dementia*. Open University Press, Buckingham.

Kitwood, T. and Bredin, K. (1992) *Person to Person: a Guide to Care of Those with Failing Mental Powers*. Gail Publications, Essex.

Morton, I. (1999) *Person-Centred Approaches to Dementia Care*. Speechmark Publishers, Oxfordshire.

Stokes, G. (2000) *Challenging Behaviour in Dementia*. Speechmark Publishers, Oxfordshire.

Thomson, P. and Mathias, P. (2000) *Lyttle's Mental Health and Disorder*, 3rd edn. Harcourt, London.

Zubin, J. and Spring, B. (1977) Vulnerability – a new view of schizophrenia. *Journal of Abnormal Psychology*, **86**(2), 103–24.

Interview question format

Theme 1: The feelings associated with dementia entering a person's life

Questions

How did you feel when you found out you had dementia?

or

How do you feel about the problems you have been having with your memory etc.?

or

How did you feel when the person was diagnosed and you were to become a carer?

- Early symptoms
- Early problems
- Telling others
- Accessing help
- Treatments

Theme 2: Emotional and practical pressures of life with these problems

Questions

How did you cope with practical and emotional pressures of life with these problems?

- House practicalities
- Socialising
- Remembering people
- Work
- Driving
- Self-care
- Feelings/mood, frustrations, effect on others

Theme 3: The past, the present, managing life and still having hope for the future

Questions

What's happening now, why and what does the future look like?

- Are you coping?
- Do others help?
- Structures/patterns/behaviours
- How do you get on with each other?
- What is the best thing going on for you just now?
- What is the most frustrating thing?
- What do you see happening next?

Contact/information sheet for respondents

Who I am

Hello,

I am Kirsty Beart. I am a teacher at Nottingham Trent University. I used to teach nursing and was a mental health nurse myself. I worked in the community with people who have dementia.

What I am doing

I am writing a book which is about people like you who are living with dementia, or caring for someone who is. So that I can make the book useful I need your input to tell me how it feels to be in this situation.

What will happen

I will ask you some key questions and then ask you to talk about whatever the questions make you think. Our chat will be recorded at the time. After, I will take out the bits I need and dispose of the tape. You will be unknown in the book unless you want to be identified. Anything you say will be used with your permission only. If you change your mind I will not use those comments.

I look forward to meeting you and hope we can work together soon.

My contact details are:

...

Index